Permission to Parent

Permission to Parent

How to Raise Your Child with Love and Limits

Robin Berman, MD

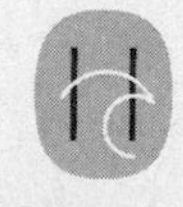

HARPER WAVE

An Imprint of HarperCollins*Publishers*
www.harperwave.com

HarperCollins books may be purchased for educational, business, or sales promotional use. For information, please e-mail the Special Markets Department at SPsales@harpercollins.com.

Library of Congress Cataloging-in-Publication Data has been applied for.

ISBN 978-0-06-227729-9

14 15 16 17 18 OV/RRD 10 9 8 7 6 5 4 3 2

To my wonderful husband, whose support for this book and support in my life are immeasurable.

To my beloved children, who raise me up.

My heart overflows with love for all of you.

Contents

Permission to Parent

Introduction

Many people spend their whole lives yearning for the loving, nurturing parents they never had. As a psychiatrist, I often feel sad when patients tearfully retell stories of what went wrong in their childhood and how deeply those moments still affect their lives. So many times I wish I could wave a magic wand, go back in time, and change those moments—before their impact becomes incorporated into who people are, how they see themselves, and how they relate to the world.

I would love this book to be your magic wand—a tool you can use to become the mother or father your children yearn for.

I love children. I always have. I babysat, was a camp counselor, was a substitute teacher, and I went to medical school to become a pediatrician or a child psychiatrist. But when I realized that healthy kids generally come from healthy parents, that's when I found my calling.

If we pay more attention to the way we parent, we can save our children so much future pain. Think of how you would have been spared if your parents were more conscious and sensitive to your needs. That is my sole intention for writing this book, to inspire parents to be their best selves, so they can be the best parents possible. I believe in preventive medicine. This book is about preventive parenting. It is my deepest wish that, in writing this, I can help someone to have a more meaningful and loving relationship with their child.

I was never a fan of old-school parenting, when children were seen and not heard, punishment was swift and corporal, hitting was the norm, and fear and shame were ways of controlling kids' behavior. Trust me, I hear stories daily of adults who were scared of their parents or fed a diet of shame. I can promise you that this is not the recipe for self-esteem.

Then this generation of children who felt neglected grew up and wanted to be more attentive than their parents had been. These new parents began to read books, go to lectures, and adopt new philosophies. Many were focused on how to foster self-esteem in their children.

I love that instinct. But, as in a game of telephone, how to actually do that got lost in translation.

Somehow children went from being seen and not heard to being the center of the universe. The whole family hierarchy collapsed, leaving children in charge, bossing their parents around. Somehow giving children self-esteem was construed to mean giving them a trophy for showing up, hovering over their every move, pouring on excessive praise, and never saying no, for fear of hurting their feelings.

In trying to constantly please our children and make them happy, we have done just the opposite. This pendulum swing has created a whole new breed of entitled, fragile kids.

The self-esteem movement backfired out of a giant misunderstanding of how real self-esteem is attained. Parents have focused too much on résumés over learning, competition over connection.

In this fast-paced culture, we have lost our perspective, our equilibrium, our internal peace. It is very difficult to offer something to our children that we ourselves don't have. The pendulum has swung too far. Children went from being neglected to being hypermanaged, while kids' real, deeper needs still remain unmet. Out of the best of intentions, we have left children too vulnerable to stress. Rates of anxiety, depression, drug use, and suicide in kids continue to rise. And I feel called to help.

Isn't there a graceful place in the middle of these parenting extremes? A hybrid approach in which we thoughtfully reflect upon what we should keep from our parents' methods, what we can learn from recent parenting trends, and what no longer serves us?

- For instance, parenting in the past was all about respecting parents; today it has become all about respecting children. How about we try mutual respect?
- Kids used to be scared of their parents; now parents are being emotionally bullied by their kids. How about setting loving limits, with you squarely at the helm?
- "You should be ashamed of yourself" was a common, damaging mantra; now we're "good job"-ing our kids to death. Let's give accurate, specific praise where it is due and delete *shame* from our vocabulary.

With all the activities we run kids to and from, and all the expectations we have of them and ourselves, family time is getting squeezed out. Parenting seems more like a profession than a relationship. But it is a relationship. A profoundly meaningful one. How we are treated as children informs much of our self-understanding. Childhood is the template for how kids learn to love and trust. It is a story that becomes deeply embedded in the fabric of our being. A strong bond with your parents builds emotional security, which allows you to be at home with yourself and to make your way in the world.

That's why I wanted to write a book about building that bond. I could write solely from my own experience—as a mother, a psychiatrist, and a parenting group leader. But I wanted to cast a broader net that captured the untapped, collective wisdom of revered teachers, respected coaches, cherished parents, beloved pediatricians, insightful therapists—and kids themselves. If we look at the commonalities from all of these sources, we find a soulful and commonsense perspective that is much simpler than we try to make it.

This book is a collection of pooled wisdom. I'm offering you my parenting Rolodex—including the people I turn to for parental inspiration—because no one should have to do this alone. It's too big a job. You're not going to get it right every time. No one does. Even if you know the right thing to do, in the heat of the moment, it's easy to react reflexively.

Sometimes we're just brought to our knees by parenting. We care so much, love so deeply, and want so badly to get it right. So I offer you this parenting village, this tapestry of experience. Take what you want, whatever resonates with you, whatever supports you, and throw the rest away.

Interviews for this book were captured by pen and paper. I scribbled quickly as wisdom poured out of these wonderful people. I did not catch every word, nor did I fact-check their stories. I tried to capture the gist of what they shared. Many stories are presented intact. In most of the anecdotes, some identifying information has been changed. A few stories are composites that took place over days or years, and were sewn together to illustrate a point more gracefully, all in the service of giving you the clearest distillation of what people had to share. Some of these stories are my own, some are from my patients, some I read about, some I heard, and others I observed.

I have learned so much from writing this book. Topping the list would be that parenting is more about raising yourself than it is about raising your child. What a great gift our children give us, if we let them: the opportunity to grow ourselves. Only then can we give our children the parents we want to be.

When you parent from your highest self, you can be of the greatest service to your children, who have entrusted you with the most precious of tasks, the task of shepherding their soul.

CHAPTER ONE

Hate Me Now, Thank Me Later

I often ask moms of this generation, "If you got on a plane and saw a four-year-old pilot in the cockpit, how safe would you feel?"

You, not your kids, fly the plane.

—Idell Natterson, PhD, psychologist

If you want to learn about parenting, head to Starbucks. You don't have to wait too long before you see a child melting down. Oh, and there he is: an adorable four-year-old boy with curly blond ringlets. Adorable, that is, until he opens his mouth to whine and negotiate for a cookie *and* chocolate milk, in spite of his mom's repeated requests to pick one or the other.

Immediately the rest of us in line transform into the parent police, secretly hoping that the mom will hold her ground, but knowing deep down that she won't. I feel as if I am rooting for the underdog in this power struggle, and her name is Mommy.

We grow more and more uncomfortable as the tantrum escalates. "I want both, you can't make me pick one. You are a mean mommy!" Everyone in line rolls their eyes at each other, and, at this point, I have to control my instinct not to intervene. I get up to the counter to order my latte and the boy smiles at me victoriously, holding his cookie *and* chocolate milk. I smile back, thinking, I will see you on my couch in twenty years.

Why is this such a common scene in today's parenting culture? Why is this generation of parents being emotionally bullied by their children? Kids are holding their parents hostage. Children used to be seen and not heard, but now they are the center of the universe. It is clear that the parenting pendulum has swung too far, and, in between these two extremes, we just might find a graceful new middle.

Parents today seem skittish about asserting their authority. I get it. These are the parents who vowed never to hit their kids as they had been hit and not to rule by an iron fist. Great instinct, but don't you think that we have gotten a little carried away? The parental power structure has gotten off-kilter. Parents today seem afraid to assume their rightful position as captain of the ship. If there is no captain, the ship will not sail, or, worse, it will sink.

I often want to take out my prescription pad and write: "You have my permission to parent."

Other physicians offer similar prescriptions.

"Parenting is an autocratic system, it is not a democracy. Children need to follow rules or else they become unruly."

—Lee Stone, MD, pediatrician

"Kids want to feel as if someone is in charge, as if someone is protecting them. Don't be afraid to assert what you think is right for your child. Don't be afraid to be in charge."

—Daphne Hirsh, MD, pediatrician

"Parenting is a benevolent dictatorship."

—Robert Landaw, MD, pediatrician

"Don't let the inmates run the asylum."

—Ken Newman, MD, psychiatrist

Today too many little inmates are clearly running the show. The truth is, if you pander to your child's worst behavior, that is exactly what you will get.

At a birthday party, a seven-year-old girl went up to the host and asked if there was going to be ice cream with the cake, and if there was chocolate chip. In a frenzy of party chaos, the host mom mumbled, "I think so."

When it was time to sing "Happy Birthday to You," Suzie began pestering the mom: "I want that ice cream," she demanded. The host mom's feathers were already ruffled; there was no "please," no "excuse me." She pulled out a tub of cookie dough ice cream and began to scoop it onto Suzie's plate.

"That is not chocolate chip," Suzie yelled, growing increasingly agitated. "You said that you had chocolate chip, and this is cookie dough. I don't like cookie dough!"

The host mom calmly explained, "I am sorry, I made a

mistake. I thought it was chocolate chip. You can either have that or a Popsicle."

Of course, you know what came next. And it is not the fantasy we all were hoping for, the one in which Suzie's mom calmly intervenes and says she understands that her child is disappointed, but that she has two choices of desserts, and the third choice is to leave the party if she can't contain herself. All the parents at the party are secretly rooting for the "leave the party" option.

"I don't want a Popsicle, and I don't like the cookie dough pieces!" Suzie screamed.

All eyes turned to Suzie's mom as she walked over to her daughter. The drama of the scene completely upstaged the birthday boy as the mother tried to cajole her child. She began with, "Oh sweetie, my love, angel, cookie dough is really good, do you want to try some?"

The child looked angry. Her mother continued, "You love Popsicles—how about an orange one?"

"No," Suzie wailed. "I want chocolate chip!" All eyes went back to Suzie's mom, our necks straining like spectators at a tennis match, hoping she could lob a winner.

Suzie's mom shocked us all. Instead of calmly asserting her parental authority, she frantically started picking out the pieces of cookie dough and putting them in her mouth, attempting to be a human pacifier. I felt as if we were being punk'd. We waited and waited. But Ashton Kutcher never came.

It is not safe for a child to have that much power. Parents seem to be tap-dancing faster and faster to try to placate their children rather than setting clear limits and asserting their authority. When you find yourself constantly bribing and negotiating, you can be sure the power structure has run amok.

The bottom line is that kids with too much power feel unsafe. Children with too much influence often become anxious because they feel like they have to control their environment, and they really don't know how. This stress triggers a cascade of toxic neurochemistry. Creating situations in which a child's developing brain is consistently bathed in the stress hormone cortisol is not a wise parenting move.

I have treated my share of anxious adults. One patient described it perfectly: "I felt sleazy being able to so easily manipulate my parents as a kid. It felt unsafe."

Parents today seem to have trouble tolerating their children's unhappy emotions. You must be able to withstand your children's disappointments and negative feelings without rushing in to fix them, or you unintentionally will be crippling your children. If you can't handle their negative feelings, how will they learn to?

Your task as a parent is to help your child self-soothe. You need to help your child build an emotional immune system. A vaccine inserts a little bacteria or a virus into your bloodstream so that you can build the immunity to fight the big one when it comes along. Think of helping your children work through negative feelings, rather than trying to fix them, as providing an emotional vaccine. You are arming them with an emotional booster for the future.

Parents who never want their kids to be upset with them, and who avoid their children's disappointment at all costs, are doing their kids a huge disservice. Good parenting can make you temporarily unpopular with your kid. Keep thinking, Hate me now, thank me later. Isn't creating a resilient adult worth enduring a few sniffles now?

Consider the message that Suzie's mother was teaching her: "If you are unhappy, whine louder to get your way. Your needs usurp all others' in the room." Fast-forward on little Suzie. Would you want to date her? Her future might be a string of one-and-dones.

By being too nice, we are actually being mean. It takes courage and some gumption to do the right thing. Take comfort in knowing that Authoritative Parenting—defined as listening to your child, encouraging independence, and giving fair and consistent consequences—yields very well-adjusted children. Spoiling a child is easier in the moment than setting limits, but it is your job to help regulate and contain your children's emotions. Emotionally wimpy parenting leads to emotionally fragile kids.

"My problem is, my kids know that my no *means* maybe.*"*

—New York mother of three

"You can't parent by the path of least resistance."

—Marc, divorced dad

"The only way to make adulthood hard is to make childhood too easy."

—Betsy Brown Braun, parenting educator and author

Parents today have way too long a fuse for bad behavior. Some moms seem to have an inordinate amount of patience for withstanding endless negotiations and tantrums, making them seem almost like Stepford Moms. A child whines and negotiates ad nauseam, and parents just keep on listening.

"I mean, how many more 'if you do that one more time's can we hear from this generation?"

—Kari, grandmother

What shocks me is how charmed parents are when their kids negotiate. They seem delighted by their kids' smarts rather than drained by their relentless lobbying. Life's simplest tasks, like going to bed or leaving the park, become fifteen-minute arguments. It is exhausting.

The power structure has capsized, and many kids are drowning. They are talking faster and faster to get their way, and it is stressful for everyone. Parents constantly ask me how to restore order.

The best way to stop a little debater in his tracks is a tool I call reverse negotiation. It works like a charm. Here is how it is done: you tell your child that negotiating will no longer be tolerated. If you are thinking that it's not that simple, you would be right. But wait, there is more—you add that when your child negotiates, not only does he not get what he was asking for, but he gets less than what he started with. Let's give it a whirl:

PARENT: Bedtime is at eight.

CHILD: I want to stay up until eight thirty.

PARENT: No, it's eight.
CHILD: I want to stay up later.
PARENT: Now bedtime is seven forty-five.
CHILD: Fine, I'll take eight.
PARENT: Now bedtime is at seven thirty.

You must stick to this revised bedtime. Cement it in, no parental trade-backs. Don't be the parent who cried wolf. Aaaah . . . Silence. All is quiet, all is well. It is as if suddenly you turned off the music on a grating radio station. If you really follow through, the little debater will vanish, and in his place will be a lovely child, snuggled in his cozy pajamas and ready for bed. Poof! Magically, the endless "if you do that one more time" tune is no longer playing in your head.

"Sometimes love says no."

—Marianne Williamson, spiritual leader, author

Ways to Think about No. Shrink-Tested and Mother-Approved

No.
No is a complete sentence.
No, that's my final answer.
No does not begin a negotiation.
No cannot mean "maybe."

CENTER OF THE UNIVERSE

Let's first be clear what your job as parent is not: grande-size playdate, entertainment center in 3-D, and, most of all, human pacifier. If you are catering to your child's every whim, you could be paving the way for a very entitled child who lacks empathy. Let's step back for a moment and think of the message we are sending to the children who are having tantrums at Starbucks or the birthday party. We are basically saying to them, Whine louder, throw a bigger fit, and you will have a cookie and chocolate milk to go with your vanilla ice cream, now that all the pieces of cookie dough have been picked out!

Teaching children empathy and that the world does not revolve around them are pretty great life lessons.

I would have loved to whisper a play-by-play in Suzie's mom's ears:

Step 1: Take a moment to calm yourself first.
Step 2: Acknowledge the feeling. "I know that you are disappointed."
Step 3: Set the limit. "It is not OK to act like this."
Step 4: Give an opportunity to self-regulate. "You can pick one of these two desserts."
Step 5: State a firm consequence. "If you can't control your behavior, we are going to leave the party."
Step 6: Follow through. Shock the parent police and actually leave. Thunderous applause will erupt.

"You have to be willing to leave the party. If your kid is acting up, you have to pull the plug. You have to let a child

know that your threats aren't empty. You would earn some cool points with the other moms if you threaten to leave and actually follow through."

—Mother of three

What Suzie needed were some clear limits that it is *not* OK to be demanding and bully people to get your needs met. She had to learn how to handle the disappointment of not getting exactly what she wanted and how to be flexible and compromise. Her mom should have tolerated her daughter's disappointment without rushing in to fix it.

Always keep your eye on the message: What am I teaching my child? In the throes of a conflict, see if you can take a deep breath, push pause, and reflect. Now push fast-forward: Am I helping to foster the qualities in my child that I value? Is how I am reacting now helpful in the long run or am I just throwing a barking dog a bone? Had Suzie's mom properly disciplined her child, that would have been the sweetest and most lasting lesson.

Your parenting should not be guided by your children's reactions. That's the wrong compass. You are wiser, older, and have better judgment. Don't let them wear you down and don't let their escalating agitation fuel yours.

"My daughter yelled one day, 'Just because I ask, doesn't mean that you have to say yes. Just say no, Mom.' I was mortified!"

—Mother of one

We are clearly seeing a generation of more entitled kids. On her first day at work, a babysitter asked the mom for instructions in caring for her seven-year-old son. The reply: "Let him be the boss and you'll have an easy day." The day might be easier for the sitter, but I can assure you life will be rougher for the boy. That same afternoon, the babysitter told him that he had to pick up his toys. He retorted, "I am going to tell my mom and she is going to fire you."

It is unbecoming—no, that is too PC—it is *obnoxious* for a child to have that much power. This boy's attitude is so out of whack with reality. And as he grows, that overdeveloped sense of importance will be disruptive in school and unappealing to potential employers. Learning the hierarchy at home enables children to respect the hierarchy of school, workplaces, and life in general.

One way to make children understand they are not entitled to everything is to say no to things they want but clearly don't need.

A mom did battle over a bathing suit in Bloomingdale's. Her thirteen-year-old was lobbying hard for a designer suit. The mom took one look at the price and said no. She explained: "I am not buying you an expensive bathing suit that you will quickly outgrow."

He begged and grew upset when she wouldn't budge. "I don't understand why you will not buy that for me. You can afford it."

She responded: "I know I can afford it, but I don't value it. You can sue me one day for teaching you values." The boy replied, "OK, you win." You have to be willing to hold your ground, to follow through and do what is right for your child, not what is easier in the moment.

Following through some times but not others spells disaster. In psychiatry we call this variable reinforcement, which means that a response is reinforced in an unpredictable manner. Gambling is a great example. You put a coin in a slot machine and sometimes you will hit the jackpot, but many times you won't, and you keep coming back just in case. Variable reinforcement can keep us stuck in bad behaviors. If your child feels that your threats are empty and that every once in a while you might follow through, it will be very hard to discipline effectively. If you say no, but only enforce it every fifth time, your words mean nothing.

Kids learn best with consistent follow-through, what we call a fixed ratio. They learn to trust that you do what you say and say what you mean. If you don't follow through, you can seem unreliable in your child's eyes. How we reinforce behavior has a dramatic effect on how our children act, respond, and ultimately behave. Discipline works best when it is consistent. It is amazing how quickly you can turn behavior around with reliable follow-through.

NO HITTING ALLOWED

The most shocking thing in parenting today is watching children hit their parents. Unfortunately, it is not that uncommon. But it is outrageous and unacceptable.

It was equally outrageous for parents of generations past to hit their kids. Parents should never use physical punishment, and there are no exceptions to this rule. You are teaching a child, by bad example, that physical violence is a way to solve problems. You are modeling out-of-control behavior yourself.

Let's check out the message: My kid is acting up, so I am

going to slug him and teach him that when he is feeling upset, just go punch someone!" This is what they know, this is what you have taught them. Yes, you may get immediate obedience in the short run, but you also may get a litany of long-term damage. Research shows that kids who are hit become less likely to comply, more likely to be physically aggressive, and increasingly vulnerable to substance abuse and mental health issues. "I was hit and I turned out fine" is a common, but lousy, rationalization. Memories of being hit plague lots of adults. Just because kids have been hit for centuries does not make it right or a valid teaching tool.

Nor is it right, in today's inverted power structure, for kids to hit their parents.

Today's crazy message is: "You're upset, go ahead and give me a good slap across the face." You are literally and figuratively giving your child the upper hand—a hand that we now know no one should raise.

At the park, a mom was chatting with some other moms, and told her four-year-old daughter that they needed to leave in five minutes. The girl pitched a fit and whined to stay longer. After the mom said they couldn't, the girl slapped her across the face. The embarrassed mom laughed nervously and continued talking to the other moms.

The mom squad looked on, shocked and horrified. They should have been. When kids think it is OK to slug Mom or Dad, all respect is lost.

A classroom needs a teacher, a ship needs a captain, a country needs a president, and your child needs a parent. Your job is not to please your child, your job is to parent your child. Your job is to set limits and boundaries to keep your kids safe.

TMI: TOO MUCH INFORMATION

Another pendulum swing in today's parenting culture is excessive talk and excessive explanations. We've gone from "No, because I said so" to reasoning through every issue until we're blue in the face.

"This generation of parents never stops talking. Parents today don't spend time just being with their children, so they try to connect by nonstop talking. It is crazy-making for a child. Children tune out after the first few words. They just stop listening."

—Early education teacher

I observed a two-year-old on a fenced-in balcony. Mom launched into a soliloquy. "Amy, don't go so close to the edge. You could fall and you could really hurt yourself and that would be so awful. It makes me nervous when you are so close to the edge. You are making Mommy nervous. I'm going to need therapy. I don't want anything to happen to you."

TMI. The child is two! How about a simple "No, honey, that is not safe," end of story.

Make it short and sweet. Give them bite-size pieces, which are easily digestible. A parent's excessive verbiage can get tuned out—or worse, become baggage. This is a perfect example of how we can unintentionally project our stuff onto our children.

It would be nice to leave childhood without having to check bags. All doctors take the Hippocratic Oath. Parents should as well. Above all, "Do No Harm."

We need to get out of the habit of creating a laundry list of our own fears and sharing them with our children. Do some verbal clutter-clearing before you speak. Children's brains are developing daily. Let's not fill them with unnecessary information, white noise, or worse, our own anxiety.

Slow down, take a deep breath, and give yourself a moment before you speak. Edit out what your child does not need to hear. Less is clearly more.

"There is way too much talking in this generation. Too much talking weakens your position as the person in charge. Kids feel unsafe."

—Midwestern therapist

"Parents today talk too much. It overwhelms a child."

—Phyllis Klein, early childhood educator

TOO MANY CHOICES

A point that closely dovetails with talking too much is giving children too many choices. This also tilts the balance of power and can overwhelm a child. Parents are now looking to kids to make decisions and, in doing so, reverse the power structure that is intrinsic to the family unit.

"With the exception of the imperial offspring of the Ming dynasty . . . contemporary American kids may represent the most indulged young people in the history of the

world. . . . They've also been granted unprecedented authority."

—Elizabeth Kolbert, "Spoiled Rotten," *The New Yorker*

It is burdensome and stressful for a child to have to make too many daily choices. I watched in shock as a mom asked her five-year-old daughter about the mother's future employment opportunities. "Do you think that Mommy should take the new job at the bank or keep my old job?"

Overload alert! Kids don't have the brain capacity for those big decisions. Kids' frontal lobes, where critical thinking resides, are still in the very early stages of development. The frontal lobe will not be fully formed until they are well into their twenties. Hence our tiny progeny do not have the neurological capacity to make decisions for us. The girl looked at her mom and said, "Beats me." Well put.

Empowering kids to make choices has to be age appropriate. "Do you want chicken or pasta?" is fine for a five-year-old girl. But asking her to weigh in on the bank job is absurd.

TOLERATING UNPOPULARITY

"Parents today are befriending their kids rather than taking their position of authority. Kids today are looking for leadership. It is nice to look up to someone bigger, stronger, and wiser than you."

—Ellen Basian, PhD, psychologist

Being your children's friend puts you on an equal playing field. The problem is, the playing field should not be equal. If we befriend our children, we are tipping the balance of power once again. If you are a friend and not a parent, then your child is left an orphan. Psychologist and author Wendy Mogel gets right to the heart of it: "Your children don't need two more tall friends. They have their own friends, all of whom are cooler than you. What they need are parents."

As a psychiatrist, I often hear from patients who longed for their parents to step up. One of my patients, Jill, had a mom who desperately wanted to be cool. She would serve alcohol to Jill's friends when they were underage, blast her daughter's favorite music while driving in the car, and dress to look hip. The mom was taken aback when Jill, by then twenty-five, asked her to join us in my office for a therapy session.

The mom began, "Jill, you are my best friend and you have always been since you were a little girl; I don't understand what went wrong."

Jill looked at her mom with tears in her eyes and said, "Mom, you tried so hard to be my friend. I have a lot of friends, but you only get one mother. I did not want your friendship, I wanted your mothering."

This point cannot be overstated. Children need and want parents. If done right, parenting will make you periodically unpopular. Take your lead from great presidents, like Abraham Lincoln. Look how kind history is to presidents who take a firm stand on doing what is right, even though it might mean being very unpopular at the time.

One great dad learned how limits make children feel safe. His son had lost his mom when he was a toddler. Jay had never known the love of an adoring mother, and, as a result, his father felt terrible and spoiled him. His father never gave him any consequences for bad behavior.

Ten-year-old Jay pitched a fit in a video store. He wanted to see a PG-13 movie that his father deemed inappropriate. Jay had a tantrum, a true fit replete with kicking and screaming on the floor. I had been working with his father on setting limits and sticking to them, but until this point, he had not had the courage to implement them. Finally the father'd had enough and calmly told Jay that they were going home without a video. Jay cried all the way home. About an hour later, the boy seemed euphoric, laughing and joking with his dad. Jay turned to his father and asked, "If I didn't get my video, why do I feel so happy?"

"Rules give kids comfort and confidence."

—Judy Mansfield, elementary school teacher

"Discipline and boundaries are a way of loving your child."

—Mother of two

You must do what you know deep down to be right, even if it means tolerating a brief drop in your poll numbers. Children are not supposed to understand all your motivations. You are the one with experience, wisdom, and perspective—a perspective that kids just do not have.

We need to be able to hold a loving space for our child's anger, hurt feelings, and disappointments. We need to stay the course in the throes of our kid's stormy emotions. Go ahead, cut loose, free yourself from fears of being the bad guy.

Tolerate disapproval today and I can assure you that history will be kind to you.

"When I was a boy of fourteen, my father was so ignorant, I could hardly stand to have the old man around. But when I got to be twenty-one, I was astonished by how much he learned in seven years."

—Mark Twain

Shrink Notes

Hate Me Now, Thank Me Later

1. Parenting is a benevolent dictatorship. Rules make kids feel safe.
2. Don't be emotionally bullied by your child. Emotionally wimpy parenting leads to emotionally fragile kids.
3. A child who has too much power often becomes anxious.
4. Catering to your child's every whim can lead to a child who is self-centered and lacks resilience.
5. Look long-term at a child who hasn't faced consequences for behavior and, therefore, never learned accountability: Would you want to date this person as an adult?
6. If you say "If you do that one more time," mean it. Consistent follow-through is essential for a child's emotional safety and your sanity.
7. Keep your eye on the long-term goal of raising a lovely child. Remember your mantra: hate me now, thank me later.
8. Talk less, give fewer choices, keep it simple. Less is clearly more.
9. When you say no, mean it.
10. Reverse negotiate. The more they argue, the less they get. It works like a charm.

CHAPTER TWO

The Strength of the Bond

We do not write the story of childhood with a dry-erase board, we write with a permanent Sharpie.

—Sue Enquist, Hall of Fame softball player and coach

Years ago I worked with a seventy-five-year-old widower who was struggling with his return to dating after a long and loving marriage. In talking about his current relationship, he brought up the way his mother had treated him as a child. Then a lightbulb went off, and he asked me: "Why is it that I have been alive for seventy-five years, and I keep talking about the first eighteen?"

Because the first eighteen are when you learn to love. Your parents are your first and most formative relationship. This connection is the stuff that grows children into well-adjusted adults. Or not. The devastating, lasting effect of a weak parent-child bond is a common denominator in the lives of many of my patients.

A strong parent-child connection is the most crucial ingredient to self-esteem. How you feel loved as a child has a huge impact on how you see yourself, relate to the world, and give and receive love. How you are treated as a child informs your identity.

The long-term effect of missing out on a safe and secure bond is so powerful that it can lead to feelings of being disconnected or unworthy. Probably the most common refrain therapists hear, no matter how much their patients accomplish, is: "It is hard for me to receive love. Deep down, I still wonder if I am really lovable. I feel lonely and empty." Without help, those who did not receive unconditional love may turn to love imposters such as food, alcohol, material acquisitions, and so forth.

On the other hand, kids who have loving connections to their parents—or, as shrinks say, who are securely attached—have an emotional tank that is full. This kind of bond fuels them for a lifetime of healthy relationships, first with themselves and then with others.

Most parents want to create that attachment, not drive their children into therapy. The vast majority of parenting mistakes are not malicious, but unconscious. We need to start parenting more consciously.

"Loving your child is an instinct. Good parenting is a teachable skill."

—Harvey Karp, MD, pediatrician and author

Today parents are consciously trying to be more involved, but are we involved in the right way? Or are we trying so hard to be good at parenting that we miss the very essence of it: a loving bond?

Lasting bonds are forged through a combination of love, limits, and time. That's the recipe for family peace.

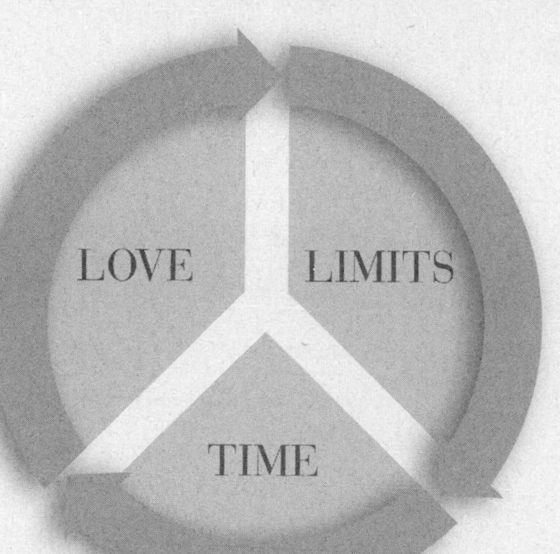

LOVE

"My parents showered me with love. I know that my confidence today stems from all of that love."

—David, University of Chicago graduate student

Unconditional love is the single greatest gift you can give to your child. Knowing that we are lovable, regardless of what we achieve or how we behave, is the crux of self-esteem.

At thirteen, Bobby was already a competitive pitcher. At

the end of the season, he was on the mound with the bases loaded and needed to strike out the next batter to win the league championship. All eyes were on Bobby as he threw ball after ball. He ended up walking the batter and losing the game for his team. He was devastated and cried all the way home, then cried himself to sleep.

The next morning he found a note his father had slipped under the door: "Dear Bobby, you will always be my MVP."

Two years later, a tearful Bobby clutched that note as he gave his father's eulogy. Because of it, he knew he would always feel loved. Because of it, his father would always be his hero.

Parenting is a true hero's journey, a love affair of epic proportions, one that lasts a lifetime and even longer. You are the author of this love story, writing and starring in it daily.

When I was in medical school, I cared for a seventy-year-old woman with cancer. After examining her and giving her some pain medication, I asked if there was anything else that she needed. I will never forget her answer: "Yes, I really need my mom."

Her mom had passed away twenty years earlier, and yet the very memory of her mother brought her great comfort. How lucky to have had that kind of parent.

That is what we are aiming for, an internalized, compassionate parent whom children carry in their heads and hearts throughout their lives. Creating that secure sense of love is the key to great parenting. A secure attachment forms when parents are consistently responsive and sensitive to the needs of their children. Such a bond is the ultimate in psychological padding: it offers a lifetime of buffering and creates emotional resilience. This tender and loving bond informs who your child will become. All great parenting has, as its foundation, a secure attachment. It's like psychic cement. With this bond, parents build an emotional house of bricks, not straw, that can weather life's inevitable huffs and puffs.

Love lays that strong foundation. To be truly seen and known—and adored because of it—is the highest form of romance.

"It is all about the connection. I want my daughter to feel how much I love her. I slow it down, I get low, I sit on the floor. I meet her where she is. I don't parent from above. I want to reach her, eye to eye, soul to soul."

—Father of three

Reaching your child and making that connection is everything. Sometimes, if you listen, you can hear even when there are no words.

During my residency, I spent six months on the pediatric floors. The pediatricians would meet and divide up the patients for the night. "Who wants death watch?" the senior resident asked callously. "She only has a few more days."

With a heavy heart, I listened to the report of an eight-year-old girl who had become mute two years before, when both parents died from AIDS. Now dying from the same disease, she was in the hospital alone. At 3:00 A.M., I poked my head in to check on her. She was so small and frail. She lay awake, staring at the ceiling. I introduced myself. Her eyes did not move to meet mine. I started to fumble through her chart, knowing deep down it was pointless. I knew my job was to examine her and check her vital signs. But the girl continued to stare at the ceiling in silence as I struggled to fit the blood pressure cuff around her bony arm. Her skin was cracking and dry, her bones showed through her emaciated body. I felt helpless and disconnected.

So I put aside my futile doctor duties. I reached for a bottle of lotion. I rubbed it all over her cracked heels and legs. When I reached for her hand, her gaze met mine for the first time. Maintaining that eye contact, I continued to massage her in silence for the next thirty minutes. When I put my hand on the door to leave, I heard a little voice say, "Thank you." I wept on the way back to my on-call room. The next morning on rounds, I learned that she had passed away at 5:00 A.M. I felt so grateful for our connection, however small, however brief.

We all yearn to feel deeply connected. Every child wants to be truly known and cherished.

Sometimes finding the keys to that connection requires a little detective work. In medical school a common mantra was "Listen to the patient, they will tell you the diagnosis." If you truly listen to your children, they will tell you who they are.

"A good parent understands the mystery of their child. They put the puzzle pieces and clues together to see who is in front of them—not who they want, but who is really there."

—Jonah, ten

Parents who remain curious and open will best be able to navigate the changing landscape that is childhood. They will continually try to understand their child, even when it's challenging—as it is when your child turns out to be different from what you imagined. We have to let go of our own agenda and expectations.

"I was a college athlete. I come from a long line of athletes. My son loves art. Go figure. I always pictured having a son who would watch football with me and throw a ball around in the backyard. Instead we spent a lot of Sundays at Michaels art supplies. I would watch his eyes light up as he dreamed up his next project. I guess that is what being a good dad is all about, seeing your kid for who he really is, and then finding a way to love him for exactly that."

—Midwestern dad

Bravo, Dad. Let go of judgment until you truly understand—your kid, the situation, and how he or she sees it. Just listening makes your child feel loved.

"The first duty of love is to listen."

—Paul Tillich, Christian philosopher

"Sometimes we forget to listen to our children. Yet listening can be very powerful. I think children, like adults, have a very strong need to be truly heard—not only heard for what they are saying on the surface, but for the feelings behind their words."

—Laura Carlin, blogger and author

Hearing the meaning behind words takes careful active listening. Kids don't always need you to fix the problem, much less to lecture, but they do need you to listen. Don't underestimate the value of listening without judgment. Really being heard and understood defuses big emotions and makes us feel comforted and connected.

Sometimes you have to set aside the small stuff that blocks connection. A mom was in the basement cleaning out toys to give to charity. She came upon a chess set with giant pieces, but a pawn was missing its bottom stand. The mom told her daughter, Ally, that they couldn't give away an incomplete set. Mom went back to her sorting, but Ally was determined to give a whole chess set to someone.

Twenty minutes later, an excited Ally exclaimed, "Look, I fixed it!" Mom turned around to see both Ally and a white couch cushion covered in black paint. Ally had glued a wood block to make a new stand and had painted it black to match the pawn. Mom was so focused on the mess that she almost missed Ally's joy at being resourceful and helpful.

"Oh, no, my couch . . ." Mom started to stammer. She saw the light fading from her daughter's eyes. Mom had to think like a chess player, two moves ahead, calming down and not squashing her daughter's enthusiasm.

"Wow, that was so clever. Someone is going to be so happy to get that chess set now that you have fixed it," she said.

By checking herself and seeing what her daughter saw, this mom did not let a little paint break a big connection. Later she was able to calmly remind Ally to lay down newspaper the next time she wanted to paint. Now, that is how the game of parenting is played.

"Our job as parents is to accurately reflect our children's experience, not our own."

—Catherine Birndorf, MD, psychiatrist and author

Sometimes we miss the point (in this example, the child's kindness) because of our own priorities (in Mom's case, an orderly house). But if you can see your child's pure experience without projecting your own stuff onto it, you will connect with their truest self.

Once you recognize your children's feelings, it's vital for you to validate them.

"I have noticed that the boys who cry the most when they are hurt have parents who always said, 'You're fine, get up, that didn't really hurt.' I think that if the mom had just hugged them, their crying would have stopped a long time ago."

—Fourth-grade boy

This wise boy is really saying that if parents are more compassionate, instead of dismissing their children's feelings, kids would pass through these phases sooner. From a psychiatrist's standpoint, minimizing children's feelings never makes them go away. It just leaves the child's needs unmet, what we call empathic failure.

When children are hurt, they need to know they have a safe parent to go to for comfort. The basics of love and comfort allow a child to depend on you. It is only through that dependence that they learn the skills to be independent. When dependency needs are not met, they keep returning in adulthood. (Think arrested development.)

Sensitive, responsive parents do quite a balancing act. They help their children manage strong emotions by knowing when to let a child work through frustration and disappointment, which increases resiliency. Today's parents are confused; they think hovering builds a secure attachment. But hovering and micromanaging are different from being an attuned parent.

Hovering/helicopter parent	**Attuned parent/secure attachment**
Intrusive, leading with anxiety, making child nervous.	Responsive, reflective, sensitive, with a calmness that is soothing to the child.
Rushes to fix or do the child's work instead of letting child work things out on his own. Gives the child a covert message: "You need me. You can't do it alone."	Gives child breathing room to figure things out; encourages with message that "you can do it."
Human emotional rip cord.	Balances when to hold and when to fold.
Bubble wraps kids, creating psychological dependence that holds them back in the real world.	Helps kids build strong psychological padding that creates a secure base, which fosters independence.

Forming a strong, secure bond is not small stuff. It is everything. Children will carry it with them for the rest of their lives. Love freely, madly, deeply. Hug, kiss, cuddle, laugh, play. Be demonstrative. Tell your children how much you love them. If you aren't your kid's biggest fan, who will be?

Remember, childhood's greatest legacy is how we felt loved.

LIMITS

While unconditional love is at the core of all great parenting, loving your child does not mean unconditional acceptance of behavior. As we saw in chapter one, kids feel safer when they have a parent firmly in charge.

"It is a great disservice to a child not to set clear and loving guidelines."

—Beth Ekre, North Dakota Teacher of the Year

Remember: all feelings are welcome; all behaviors are not. Once guidelines are set, you have to enforce them consistently. Not following through with kids is like not finishing an antibiotic. One grows resistant bacteria, the other resistant kids.

But in this new age of parenting, we seem ambivalent about the concept of discipline. Maybe it is because we have confused being in charge with the harsh disciplinarians of generations past. These two are distinct. Discipline done right fosters self-esteem, whereas harsh or shaming discipline erodes self-esteem.

There is never a time when screaming, shaming, or hitting a child is justified. True discipline does not involve any of those things. It is an opportunity to teach your child. In fact, *discipline* means "to teach."

Twelve-year-old Matthew was a tournament tennis player.

His parents went to watch their son in the semifinals. Matthew was very agitated on the court. As his frustration increased, his sportsmanship began to nosedive. Matthew became so upset that after losing a critical point, he threw his racket.

Matthew's dad walked on the court and calmly told his son that he was going to have to forfeit the match. The son began to cry and begged his father to let him continue the game, but his father stayed the course.

"I know that this is very upsetting for you, but throwing your racket is not OK," Dad continued. "We care more about sportsmanship than we do about winning. I have given you two warnings about your body language and your attitude on the court, and now you're going to forfeit the match. I feel so bad that you have to forfeit."

The dad did not yell or berate his child in any way. In fact, he empathized with his son's plight, and he took Matthew's behavior as an opportunity to teach him a life lesson. Having a boundary, and a firm consequence when the child crosses the line, creates accountability. That in turn empowers children to police their own sense of right and wrong.

The key to setting effective limits is to let your child know that his or her feelings are valid, even empathized with, but the limit remains. This was a turning point for Matthew. He talks today with pride about his dad's intervention. Matthew went on to win sportsmanship awards in both high school and college.

"Sometimes a child's really bad choice can lead to a really great defining moment."

—Educator

This father's parenting was exemplary. His empathy for his child and calm delivery created an alliance and strengthened their bond. He loved his kid right through the lesson. He was a calm, clear leader. He did not react with anger or rage. He did not shame his child.

What if a furious father had run out on the court, screaming at his son, "You should be ashamed of yourself," "You have humiliated me," "How dare you," etc., etc.? This type of intervention just does not work. You might control the behavior in the short run, but all you are really doing is eroding the parent-child bond in the long run.

Shaming is hard to shake. Trust me on this one. It's toxic! It's just destructive noise that chips away at a developing self. That's not what parents are trying to do when they discipline their kids. But many times in my office, I have heard adults persistently repeat these comments to themselves with a deep sense of shame. The harmful words are no longer being said by the parents; they are now the negative narration in the child's head. Shaming becomes internalized self-hatred.

"My mom constantly called me lazy when I was growing up. Now, no matter how hard I work or how much I achieve, I think I'm lazy."

—Tales from the couch

"Every time I sang as a child, my mother told me I had a terrible voice and should never sing loudly. Would you believe to this day I still mouth 'Happy Birthday'?"

—Alison, forty-two

"When I was little, my mom used to tell me that I had fat feet. I am always self-conscious when I wear sandals, and I am seventy-three."

—Grandmother

It's hard to cast off the messages of childhood and to silence the voice that is now on automatic replay.

The way you talk to your kids is the way that they will talk to themselves. You are the voice in your child's head.

The effect of shaming words can't be overstated. *You are lazy, you're selfish, you're sneaky* gets programmed into your offspring's head and directly into their feelings of self-worth. Whether talking to your toddler, teen, or emerging adult, remember that your words will echo for years—and likely get passed down to your grandkids.

I recently walked into a basketball practice, and as I stepped one foot into the gym, I heard a mother berating her son: "Move it, you're so slow. What is wrong with you? What is your problem?"

I must not have hidden my shock. The mom said, "Oh, sorry, I wasn't talking to you!"

I laughed and answered, "Oh, that's a relief! That's just how you talk to your *son*!"

Someone who screams at her child is not an involved parent but an unenlightened parent. Can you imagine what is already programmed into this nine-year-old boy's head?

Parents today are hypervigilant about the wrong things. The value of going to every game is lost when you spend that time tearing down your child. Using harsh words to coach basketball moves is shortsighted. Loving through carefully chosen language pays much bigger psychological dividends. Nothing will line up future success more than having your child internalize a loving and compassionate voice instead of a harsh and punitive one.

"Would you feed your kids junk food all day long? So don't feed them junky thoughts."

—Family therapist

This is a tall order, I know. Parenting presents you with so many unpredictable moments that shock you. When we don't take time to think about how to respond, we revert back to the old way we were parented. Words fly out of our mouths before we have a chance to filter them.

If it was someone else's kid on the court throwing the racket, we would not feel as reactive. But with our own child, love makes us irrational, and we go from zero to irate in two seconds. Emotions hijack our best judgment and can lead to a delivery that we are not proud of. It is easy in the heat of the moment to react with anger, shame, or blame.

The classic example is parents screaming at their kids to calm down. We can either model calmness or we will match their agitation tantrum for tantrum. So breathe, and think, before you speak.

Think of choosing language as a way of loving your child! Language can unite, or language can divide. Mindful parenting is the ultimate in damage control. Think of how you would have been spared had your parents chosen their words with more care.

The most stellar parents and teachers I interviewed all

understand this essential secret: choosing words with grace is the most underrated tool in creating a strong parent-child bond—or any healthy relationship, really. In order to engage your child's highest self, you have to talk to his or her highest self.

"If I can't reach my child, I need to approach them with more care and different words."

—Judy Mansfield, California teacher

"When emotions are charged, and a child is frustrated, and when real learning is at a premium, words should be highly choreographed."

—College coach

If words are choreography, delivery is music. And if the volume is turned too high, kids will just tune out.

"When my mom screams so loud, I can never hear her words, only the screaming. First I feel scared, then sad. . . . Sometimes I wish that I had a different mom."

—Tales from the couch

Rage and punishment may control behavior in the short run. Kids who are scared of their parents might appear submissive and even well behaved. But I assure you that intimidation as a means of control chips away at the foundation of the child's self-esteem and paves the way for defenses to be built. The child's real self goes underground. My job as a psychiatrist is to chisel away at those defenses and re-parent in a safer way.

So please help put me out of business. Let's not fire the verbal arrows that make our kids build walls around their hearts. Instead of unleashing sharp words, try to keep them to yourself. We have an opportunity in each moment to give or to take, to add or subtract to our kids' lives. Conscious choices with our words can edit a frustrated inner monologue into a more constructive dialogue. Practice filtering your thoughts so you don't say hurtful words that can't be taken back.

In other words, grow the muscles that will let you be *reflective*, not *reflexive*. This takes patience, practice, and commitment. But I can assure you it is so worth it. When you are calm and rational, you can set limits with love.

"When I am on overload and my kids are acting up, I give myself a time-out. I give myself a beat. I tell my girls that I will be right back. I sit on my bed and breathe. I give myself a moment so that I can calm down and feel more balanced."

—Stay-at-home dad

That simple act has a profound effect. Exciting neuroscience research shows that if we parents can model calmness when our emotions are running high, we teach our kids to manage their emotions—what doctors call affect regulation. Affect regulation, in turn, lays down neurological pathways for a more resilient brain. In the prefrontal cortex, the brain governs decision making, attention, problem solving, and judgment. When emotions run high, the brain does not work as well. But if you stop to pause and calm your emotions, rational thought kicks back in. That takes practice to learn, and watching a parent do it helps children learn it, too. The brain is shaped by its experiences. Put simply, if you scream or get agitated at your kids, and your children regularly experience your uncontrolled emotions, then their brains will wire for uncontrolled emotion. But if you can parent calmly, you are literally wiring your child's brain to be calmer. Thus your parenting has profound implications for your child's brain development. That's why it is essential to regulate your own emotions and teach your children to do the same.

But here is the parenting paradox: you can't teach what you don't know. Ah, so this is why they say our children are our greatest teachers. At the heart of good parenting is a lot of self-reflection and self-discipline. If you tend to fly off the handle or be short-tempered or impatient, here is an opportunity for growth.

Look how everyone evolved in this story. Two brothers were fighting and screaming over Legos. Just when Zach went to grab a piece out of the hand of his brother, Eric, the mom intervened. "Stop that! Stop fighting!" she yelled, frustrated. But then, instead of playing the harried referee, she quieted her tone and remembered a technique used in Montessori schools.

"Boys, I have an idea," she whispered. "Let's have you sit in the peace chair to settle the fight." She placed two kids' chairs facing each other. She picked up a giant paintbrush and held it with reverence. "This is the talking peace stick," she said quietly, as if creating sacred folklore. "When you hold the stick, you may tell your side of the story. Your brother can't speak while you hold it, he can only listen. Then your brother will get a turn."

Seven-year-old Eric gently took the peace stick and explained, "I need the blue Lego to finish my ship."

Then it was five-year-old Zach's turn. His sobs softened as he began to realize he was going to be heard. "I am making a car and I really, really need the blue Lego, and there are no blue Legos left."

So Mom offered the stick back to Eric with a question.

"I see that you both want the Lego. How do you think you could work it out?"

Eric thought for a moment and lit up with excitement. "I know, we both can start over and divide up all of the blue, green, yellow, and red pieces from the beginning and start over with exactly the same amount."

Eric passed the talking stick to Zach, who managed one sentence through his tears: "I love you, Eric."

The mom said to herself, Wow, I'm shocked that actually worked!

Let's review what she did right.

- She calmed her own emotions down—we have to be the lesson before we can teach the lesson.
- She modeled a gentle tone.
- She set out clear rules for how to talk to each other.
- She gave the boys an opportunity to learn conflict resolution by empowering them to work it out themselves. They became more invested in the outcome and active participants in the problem solving.

And that's how she transformed a fight about a piece into real peace.

"Every time you are tempted to react in the same way, ask if you want to be a prisoner of the past or a pioneer of the future."

—Deepak Chopra

You are the hero or heroine of this fleeting story called childhood. How do you want to pen the tale?

Setting Limits with Love

1. Calm yourself. Check your own composure. Never discipline your child without first disciplining yourself.
2. Have empathy for your child's struggle. Be with him, not against him.
3. Teach and hold the limit with respect. No shame, no blame.

TIME

In *The Gift of an Ordinary Day*, the author Katrina Kenison writes about the preciousness of time and how quickly it passes.

> Somehow our treasured family ritual of reading together at bedtime slipped away. No one asked for stories anymore.

> Baths were replaced by showers. . . . Baseballs stopped flying in the backyard. A bedroom door that had always been open, quietly closed. . . . I missed my old world and its funny little inhabitants, those great big personalities still housed in small, sweet bodies. I missed my sons' kissable cheeks and round bellies, their unanswerable questions, their innocent faith, their sudden tears and wild, infectious giggles.

Soak it up while it is happening because it is gone too soon. Spend time. Make memories. Experience every moment you can. Give that gift to yourself and to your children.

I once read: "Kids spell love *T-I-M-E*." We need to put time into childhood—slow, present time. From a psychiatrist's standpoint, errors of omission are tough to forgive. Remember Harry Chapin's song "Cat's in the Cradle." It's hard to shake the memory and pain of absence. How we prioritize our time sends a clear message to our kids about what we value.

"I can promise you that no social engagement is as important as the one you have with your kids at home."

—Bobbi Brown, cosmetics guru, at an L.A. luncheon

We can't farm out parenting to others, or to activities and electronic distractions. Our kids need to feel our real presence in their little lives. You don't get a pass on this.

"Parenting cannot be outsourced."

—Marc Weissbluth, MD, pediatrician and author

On the first day of elementary school, Ray Michaud, a principal for thirty-six years, begins his speech to the parents: "As much as possible, clear your calendar. These are special, formative years; these are the years your kids want to be with you. Trust me; you won't want to miss them, they don't come back."

These are the years when your kids ask for one more bedtime story, for one more moment of watching them color, for you to stay in their room and snuggle one minute longer. Do.

"So here are the things I do . . . things that don't come naturally to me . . . things I could easily take a pass on, but I don't. I do these things—not because I enjoy them—but because someone very important to me does. . . .

"I watch her lip-synch Taylor Swift music videos—not because I like to hear 'We Are Never Ever Getting Back Together' ten bazillion times—but because the facial expressions she makes are indescribable, and I want to remember them when I am eighty years old."

—Rachel Macy Stafford, handsfreemama.com

In interview after interview, parents talked about how spending time makes their children feel so loved. People carry with them always the small, daily acts of love. A few extras go a long way, too.

"I was a single mom, exhausted, working full-time and raising my two kids. It was a cold winter's night, and I had just read the story Owl Moon *to my daughter.*

"'How come we never go out at night owling?' she asked.

"What went through my mind was that I am exhausted and could barely make it through reading a story about owling, let alone go out on a cold winter's night, but I decided to make a grand mommy gesture. I bundled my kids up in their winter clothes and took them in the car to chase the moon. We drove about twenty minutes until we found an open field and parked. We sat in the car, staring at the moon.

"I will never forget the feeling of being with my kids, bundled up together and gazing at the starry sky. In retrospect, I wish I had spent more nights chasing the moon."

—Midwestern mother of two

The Parenting Pendulum

Old School	*Today's Trends*	*New Middle*
Punitive dictator	Anarchy/kids rule	Benevolent leader
Harsh discipline	No discipline	Calm, clear, loving limits
Neglect	Hovering	Secure attachment
Naughty chair	Time-out	Peace chair
Shaming words	Sugarcoated speech	Choosing words with grace
Children seen and not heard	Only children are heard	Acknowledge children's feelings but maintain your leadership

Shrink Notes

The Strength of the Bond

1. You want to inspire and teach, not punish or shame.
2. Take a parental time-out. Put some space in between what's annoying you and your response.
3. Consequences teach accountability.
4. Calm, clear, consistent limits create an alliance. Setting limits thoughtfully is a way to love your child.
5. Discipline teaches children self-discipline.
6. Show empathy for your child's struggle. Empathy defuses big emotions. Remember you are on the same team, working together to grow a great child.
7. When you are calm, you teach your children that they, too, can regulate their emotions—you show them how. That grows a more resilient brain.
8. Choose language with care. Shaming words are toxic and erode children's self-confidence and self-worth.
9. How you talk to your kids is how your kids will talk to themselves. You are the voice in their heads.
10. Childhood's greatest legacy is how we felt loved.

CHAPTER THREE

Look, No Hands!

> At every step the child should be allowed to meet the real experiences of life; the thorns should never be plucked from the roses.
>
> —Ellen Key, teacher and author

The packaging instructions for childhood should read: "Handle with care," not "Fragile, will break."

Now that we've established the importance of making a deep connection, we have to remember to let our children discover their independence. Kids gain so much when they learn to do things for themselves.

Back in the day, parents would sit on the park bench while their kids played. Today you will commonly see parents on the play structure showing their kids how to play, or worse yet, fighting their kids' battles. While many parents aren't disciplining when they should, too many parents are intervening when they shouldn't.

Two four-year-old boys were on the swings, their moms pushing from behind. Max began to cry, saying that he did not like the end swing; he wanted the middle swing. Will eyed him curiously but kept pumping his legs. Max began screaming, "I want the middle swing!" As the noise became more disruptive, and the parent posse grew restless, Max's mom jumped in. But instead of addressing her child, she glared at Will's mom and snapped, "You can see that my son wants the middle swing. Can your son get off?"

Seriously? This woman's judgment was clouded by her inability to let her child experience even a modicum of disappointment. Not letting a kid suffer is not about the child's growth or development. It is actually about alleviating a parent's anxiety.

The mom's rant continued: "My child is so upset, I need your son to get off the middle swing." Clearly a parenting low moment, surreal in feel, but all too common today. No, this is not the twilight zone; this is a courtside seat at the crazy game of extreme parenting. Any referee watching parents today would constantly be yelling "Interference!" Gone are the days when moms had neither careers nor nannies, when kids played kick the can in the street and came home when the sun went down. Moms could not attend to every need and desire—and didn't. They did not hover, they did not overanalyze. Today's mothers vowed to be different.

Our intentions were honorable: we wanted to be more attentive to our kids than our parents had been to us. We wanted their feelings to be more central than ours had been to our parents. But don't you think we've gone a little overboard? We are a generation of pleaser parents, being pushed around by our own kids. The previous generation of parents was clear about the family hierarchy: I am the parent; you are the child. They wanted to be respected, whereas today's parents want to be loved. Almost the way someone romances a mate, hoping to earn affection, today's parents are doing somersaults to court their own kids. It's dizzying.

"Honor thy father and mother" makes good sense—always has, always will. What past generations were missing was a respect for the child. That's the piece that needed to be added. But instead of instilling mutual respect, we abandoned respect for parents. We have somehow confused honoring children's feelings with giving in to their every whim.

In addition, our good intentions have morphed into intrusion, hyperconcern, and one gigantic piece of bubble wrap. We are insulating against scrapes that haven't yet occurred.

It's insidious. Pick up a baby catalog and check out the real gadgets sold to baby-proof the natural flow of child development: baby knee pads, toddler helmets, and the like. Have we forgotten that children come preassembled? Toddlers' brains have natural helmets called skulls. Their tiny bodies have tons of extra padding in the form of chunky, delicious thighs. When falling does occur, they're covered. Isn't nature clever? Of course, as your child ages and starts climbing on bicycles and skateboards, helmets will become necessary. But don't worry about a few bumps and bruises when kids are toddling around.

Bruised knees and bruised feelings let children learn how to deal with life's inevitable pain. Learning from adversity is what eventually makes an adult of a child. Kids need to learn to climb little fences, so when they grow up they can scale the big ones. Children must learn to trust themselves to navigate the world.

But how can they do this if their parents keep being a human GPS? Many mothers I interviewed reported seeing moms in the sandbox taking a shovel back when one was grabbed out of their kid's hands—obliterating all opportunities for the children to learn how to work it out on their own. Who is to blame, the kids themselves? Clearly not!

Let's go back to basics and take our cue from the mother of all mothers: Mother Nature. If a mother hen tries to crack the eggshell to help her baby out, the chick dies.

Here lies a major problem with parenting today: our hovering and overinvolvement are preventing our kids from fully hatching. Just as the hen has to let the chick make its own way out of the shell, parents have to let their kids walk around without trying to prevent every fall. Our own worries and fears are wreaking havoc on our parenting—and on our children. Parents are trying to take the sharp edges out of their kids' lives. But part of life is negotiating the edge. When we remove it, we deprive children of the opportunity to practice assessing and managing risk. Pain is instructive. When kids feel physical pain, they learn to avoid dangers.

Overprotection creates psychological fragility. And if you treat children like they are fragile, they will stay fragile for life.

"Don't treat me like a feather that needs to be protected in the world!"

—Jackson, ten

That little boy is so right. Give children a little leeway. Don't panic if they fall, physically or metaphorically. Failure, like bumps and bruises, lets children learn from their mistakes. Many of our greatest legends found their footing in failure.

Let's Play Jeopardy with Some Famous Failures

From North Carolina, six foot six, cut from his high school basketball team as a freshman. He has said: "I have missed more than nine thousand shots in my career. I have lost almost three hundred games. . . . I have failed over and over and over again in my life and that is why I succeed."

Who Is . . .
Michael Jordan

Twelve publishing companies rejected her manuscript before she went on to capture the world's imagination with her stories about a wizard with a lightning scar on his forehead.

Who Is . . .
J. K. Rowling, author of the Harry Potter series

You get the picture.

Watching our children struggle with what we perceive to be difficult (and perception is the key here) can be trying. Knowing when to step in and when to hold back is one of the hardest balancing acts of parenting. But today the pendulum is swinging too often into code red. Instead of allowing mistakes and failure to be some of our kids' best teaching tools, parents today treat emotional pain and mistakes like a hot stove. We have it all wrong. Our job is not to prevent our kids from failing; it is to teach them that failure is part of the process of success.

"A person who never made a mistake never tried anything new."

—Albert Einstein

"The greatest glory in living lies not in never falling, but in rising every time we fall."

—Nelson Mandela

Failure is how kids learn perseverance. Knowing that you can bounce back from failure and disappointment teaches inner resiliency and builds true self-esteem. Real self-esteem comes from mastery—social, physical, and emotional—coupled with unconditional love.

But we've lost the crux of self-esteem—the word *self*! Instead of allowing our children to stumble their way through, we persist in micromanaging everything so that our children never feel any modicum of hurt. This is not self-esteem, this is insanity!

Let's look back at the swing set debacle. It could have been a great opportunity for the kids to learn to compromise and to handle a little disappointment. How?

Shrink-approved ending number one: the kids worked it out themselves.

Shrink-approved ending number two: Max's mom told Max that the middle swing is already taken. He learned patience, and that other people's feelings matter.

Actual ending: Will's mom, a TV actress, reluctantly pulled Will off the swing. In an attempt at an apology, Max's mom asked Will's mom for her number so the boys could have a playdate. Looking stunned, Will's mom snapped: "Your son is a brat, and if you keep parenting your kid like this, his future looks even brattier." No, this was not a line from her sitcom, but it could have been reality TV.

Instead of taking a deep breath and letting our children work through conflicts, we jump in. We need to relax and to cut our kids some slack. But that's hard to do in a zero-tolerance culture that relentlessly demands perfection. People used to understand that child development had ebbs and flows. Now the natural foibles of childhood cause anxiety and fear.

That's why we call in so many "experts." Today we have sleep-training experts, toilet-training experts, and even thumb-sucking experts.

Enter, stage left, the Bike Whisperer.

Oscar, a preschool teacher, is making bank teaching five-year-olds how to ride bikes.

According to Oscar: "Parents today are not letting go of the bike." They literally don't let go! They keep jogging, holding on to the back of the bike, looking like they are in dire need of CPR and telling their kids they're not going to let them fall.

"It cracks me up. Because the odds of not falling when you learn to ride a bike are pretty much zero," Oscar says.

The Bike Whisperer sends the nervous parents to get coffee so he can let the kids find their confidence. Their first questions? "Am I going to fall? Is it going to hurt?" Oscar shoots straight: "Yes."

That's where Oscar gets his power. He lets the kids fall, which lets them learn to steer. If the parent is in control by holding on to the bike, the child is always looking back for his balance. When Oscar lets go, the kids find their own balance, their own "locus of control," as we say in psychiatry.

By the time the parents come back, their kids are riding—down the road and right into life.

DEPENDENCY BREEDS RESENTMENT

Not letting go of the metaphorical bike, or overprotection, blocks children's emerging independence. As a result, kids don't learn to do things for themselves. That lack of self-empowerment frustrates children, who may be too young to recognize or express those feelings. So they act out.

Their bratty behavior often shocks their parents, who expect gratitude for all their efforts. But why would children be grateful when we have just made them more needy? Instead of teaching children to do for themselves, we have given them the message that when the inevitable bumps occur, Mommy and Daddy will rush to the rescue 24/7.

"Parents today swoop in over nothing to prevent their kids from suffering. If they keep it up, it looks like they will have a permanent job."

—Charlie, seventeen

That also is what's making parents exhausted and resentful. In my office and my parenting groups, countless parents have confessed the same thing: "I feel guilty that I am not enjoying my child." Parents grow weary when they have to do everything for their children. But children cannot take over even the most mundane tasks if Mommy and Daddy won't let them. It's a vicious cycle that wears parents out and frustrates children.

"Overprotective parents give the message to children that they have to be protected. Good parents protect their child from harm, but also honor their inborn need to explore and differentiate."

—Isaac Berman, PhD, psychologist

Instead of becoming happier, our kids are growing angrier and more fragile. Overparenting and overprotection have truly backfired. Kids today are not better off; they're more dependent, more risk averse, more entitled, and less resilient. And I know this is not what we were aiming for.

I observed two four-year-old girls playing Candy Land, a fun childhood game of luck in which you weave your way to the rainbow finish line. Jenny was winning the game, while Beth was looking defeated. Beth became more teary-eyed and angry at each turn. Unfortunately, her mom's anxiety rose in direct proportion to Beth's. Beth's mom overidentified with her child's pain, or, as we shrinks say, she became enmeshed. Her boundaries got blurred.

Beth's mom jumped in to rescue her kid from further emotional hurt. "Everyone is a winner at Candy Land!" she gleefully declared.

(Shrink declares, "Oh, boy!")

Little Jenny looked confused. "That is not how you play Candy Land," she said. "Someone has to lose."

Kids know there are winners and losers in games. But when parents "protect" them with lies like "Everybody wins," it not only feels disingenuous to children but also makes them question what they see with their own eyes. We don't want to be skewing their internal truth meters in the interest of making them feel better. Otherwise we just sound like Jack Nicholson in the film *A Few Good Men*: *"You can't handle the truth."*

But kids can. Parents are the ones who need to get comfortable being uncomfortable. Beth's mom needed to sit with her unease of watching her child struggle. Wrestling their way through challenges lets kids build emotional muscles and literally builds a stronger brain.

"Good parents let kids fall and stumble without becoming alarmed. They know that childhood has setbacks."

—Nat Damon, educator

Let's take another example from Mother Nature. Butterflies have to fight their way out of the cocoon. The process of beating their wings against the chrysalis strengthens the wings. If someone else breaks the chrysalis, the butterfly will never fly. Struggle precedes flight. When it is painful to watch your children be frustrated, remind yourself that their growth will depend on your willingness to let them find their way through. Think of those glorious wings!

"Parents have such a tough time seeing their kids disappointed or in emotional pain. They want to fix everything. We often don't really have the power to fix it. Honor your child's thoughts and feelings as they are, no matter how difficult."

—Julia, therapist

Whether in Candy Land or in life, every child needs to learn how to lose and to be a good sport, and most of all to tolerate frustration. I know it's harder in the moment to see your child saddened, but don't confuse your need with theirs. I know it seems easier to show your child the way, rather than back away. Good parenting starts with self-correction. Identify your own internal alarm bell, and then turn down the volume. Before you rush to a knee-jerk rescue, wait. Remember that waiting means "to pause for another to catch up, to hold back."

I know it seems counterintuitive, but your goal should be to let your child get frustrated. Kids grow when they're frustrated; they increase their psychological padding. They make connections when they process discomfort. It literally makes them more resilient.

In medical school one of our mantras was "Use it or lose it." Use your muscles and they strengthen; use your brain and it grows. PET scans and MRIs have led to an exciting new understanding of how the brain works and have proven that our brains are malleable (medically known as neuroplasticity). According to Judy Willis, MD, a leading neuroscientist, "The more we use neural circuits, the more electricity that flows through them, the greater the neuroplastic growth." Put simply, learning a new behavior, like frustration tolerance, actually shapes your child's brain for the better.

Just as true love seems to be forever engraved in the architecture of your heart, learning a new behavior changes the architecture of your brain. That should give you the strength to step back and allow your children to have the arc of their own experience. Often just being a loving presence is enough. See your child as capable of working through discomfort, then stand back and let her do it. Let her learn that she does not have to spend her life avoiding emotional hurts.

"The best way out is always through."

—Robert Frost

Anxiety comes from walking around issues and not through them. Emotional courage is not the absence of fear, but rather the ability "to feel the fear, and do it anyway."

A moving example of working through emotional pain comes from a grieving widow and her four-year-old daughter. When little Emma was three, her father was killed in a car accident. Her mother, Anne, was angry and devastated by the loss of her husband. It was so painful for both mother and daughter that after his funeral they never spoke about him. Their emotional pain continued to escalate. The newly single working mother returned home at night exhausted, and she would lose her patience quickly with her daughter. The dynamic between them became one of anger and frustration. They seemed to be growing further and further apart.

Anne enrolled in my parenting group. The group encouraged her to talk about the death of her husband with her child, but she refused, saying that it hurt too much. Weekly she would arrive at the group looking sad and worn-out. Avoiding their raw feelings was taking its toll on both mother and daughter.

The final week of the group, Anne returned looking peaceful for the first time. The group asked her what had happened. She said that Emma had asked to read a story before bed and had chosen *The Lion King*. Anne had never read it and was happy to be reading something new, when all of a sudden she realized that the father lion died.

"My instinct was to skip over the next few pages so that my daughter would not be in pain, but because of my work in the group, I read those pages to her," Anne said. "Emma began to weep. She threw her head in my lap and sobbed, 'My dad died, too, just like the Lion King!' "

Anne reported that they both wept holding each other. "As painful as it was, I felt so close to her for the first time since her dad died. I felt relieved to see Emma crying, and I felt like I was really comforting her. . . . Emma asked where her daddy was and I explained that he was in heaven. She asked if she could hug him. I told her that we could hug him in our hearts. Emma leaped up and ran to the closet and got a mitten and yardstick. She put the mitten on the yardstick and held it up high and said, 'Hi, Dad, it's me, Emma. I just wanted to give you a hug.' "

Your child will not break from emotional challenges, neither the big ones nor the little ones. In fact, hurdles are opportunities for growth.

I observed a master teacher guide two first-grade boys through a routine challenge with such joy. The boys were fighting over a book. Mrs. Freid approached them with a big smile on her face and said in a lilting southern accent, "I am so excited right now, as you boys are going to learn how to compromise."

"What is a compromise?" one boy asked, already disarmed by the teacher's enthusiasm.

"You are going to get a little of what you want, and your friend is going to get a little of what he wants, and you are going to come back and tell me how it all worked out," Mrs. Freid said. I was surprised at how readily they bought what she was selling. She did not try to solve the boys' fight over the book. Instead she gave them an opportunity to learn for themselves and grow from the experience. The boys came up with a time-sharing plan and used eenie-meenie-miney-mo to figure out who got the book first. No longer fighting, they looked very pleased with themselves.

This is where the gold is in parenting. This is how we build self-esteem. This, I can assure you, is a much sweeter lesson than making it first to the Candy Land finish line.

So are we clear? The whole helicopter-parenting thing has been a real bust with some serious ramifications. We psychiatrists are seeing a huge increase in anxiety disorders, drug dependence, and depression in kids, adolescents, and young adults. It's devastating.

Unintentionally this generation of loving parents is sending its kids off into the world with empty coping slots in their emotional toolboxes. Children are going to college and calling, texting, and Skyping their parents daily, asking them for advice on decisions that they should be making themselves. One professor told me that parents are even correcting their kids' college papers via e-mail. Who knew that college honor codes would have to include parents? An electronic leash today is pulling young adults back, just when they need to run free.

The coolest part of college used to be the feeling of being independent and capable of making your own decisions. College is the bridge from home to real life. Learning self-reliance is a developmental stage you can't just skip. We know what Oscar would say: "Let go of the darn bike!" Teach children that it is OK to fall and that they are quite capable of surviving the bruises.

"Self-esteem has to be learned and earned through meeting challenges. It is not something a parent can hand a child. It's an inside job."

—Vivien Burt, MD, PhD, psychiatrist

GOOD OLD-FASHIONED ELBOW GREASE

One way to teach kids what they're capable of is to give them work to do. Many parents I interviewed lamented the lost work ethic of this generation. Too often, today's babysitter isn't embarrassed if you come home to find her texting, the kids still up, and the dishes not done. And she's looking for her money. The nerve!

That's another pendulum shift. A lot of young people today lack an understanding of hard work. Many business executives I interviewed echoed the same complaint: "Kids today think they are too special to start at the bottom." Kids think that they can start where we left off, and they're no longer willing to pour coffee or start in the mailroom. They think they can skip over the hard work that is essential to success.

"This generation lacks oomph. They don't want to work their way up. From the beginning, their parents put them on a pedestal. They have nothing left to reach for."

—Janice, psychologist

In fact, the Millennial Generation feels so entitled, the National Institutes of Health reports that 40 percent believe they should be promoted every two years, regardless of how hard they work or how well they perform.

One easy way to prevent such an attitude is to teach kids to work from the start. Parents are so focused on academic and athletic achievement that they forget to make kids accountable and good citizens at home. They have not required them to do household chores or to get summer jobs. Being accountable to a parent or a boss at a young age creates a sense of responsibility. Being on your own at a job teaches you to show up, have a good attitude, and work hard. That fosters self-confidence, which only multiplies.

"The harder you work, the luckier you get."

—Gary Player, Hall of Fame golfer

Today's hyperfunctioning parents meet many of their kids' emotional and material needs and in doing so take hunger out of the equation. But if you take hunger out of the equation, then you deprive your kids of the opportunity to long for something, as well as the satisfaction of earning it. If they feel too satiated, they become complacent. Hunger fuels drive.

A business executive traced his road to success back to his boyhood days in India. In spite of owning five cars, his father made him take the bus to his summer job. The bus stopped multiple times and added an extra hour to the young man's commute. Sitting on a packed bus through stifling heat gave him the motivation to work to buy a car the following summer. Though the story might sound a little draconian, the executive credits a measure of his success back to his frustrating experience of riding that bus.

Another dad raised two sons who, combined, attended Harvard, Dartmouth, the University of Pennsylvania, and the University of Chicago. Now both are thriving in their careers and family lives. I asked the father how he thought his two sons had become so motivated. Without missing a beat he replied, "It was so easy. I let hard work teach the lesson. Every summer I would scour the want ads for the hardest, most physically taxing summer jobs that I could find that paid minimum wage. One summer I had my son Dan loading heavy boxes onto a truck from morning until night. When he asked me to buy him a pair of basketball sneakers, I would ask him how many hours he thought that he would have to work to be able to pay for the shoes."

Dan, who went on to become a cancer surgeon, said, "Medical school was easy in comparison."

The road to success is often paved with overcrowded buses and heavy crates that need loading. Ironically, not bubble wrapping the road often leads to a smoother ride. Let's leave the bubble wrap for presents and give our kids a true gift, the gift of self-reliance.

FALSE PRAISE

"I wanted my kids to feel good about themselves. I thought I could manufacture it with exaggerated praise, but that strategy backfired. . . . Instead of fueling confidence, I fueled entitlement."

—Paula, grandmother

"False praise is like overblowing a balloon: popping is inevitable."

—Roger, father

Parents today think that they can pass out self-esteem like dessert. They sprinkle it on their children, thinking that it is the essential spice in the recipe for cooking secure kids. Research shows that the inverse is true. The *-est* words can be harmful on many levels. The "You are the fastest/smartest" type of feedback leaves kids no incentive for growth and undermines development. A landmark study by the psychologist Carol Dweck shows that overpraised kids are less resilient and more risk averse. According to Dweck, "If praise is not handled properly, it can become a negative force, a kind of drug that, rather than strengthening students, makes them passive and dependent on the opinion of others."

From a shrink's perspective, constant praise does not foster self-esteem: being known does. Constant praise instead fosters a neediness for more praise and creates an extremely self-conscious child. The excessively praised child may be prone to exaggerate accomplishments, or, on the flip side, be overly self-critical.

Praise works best when it is specific, and when you praise the effort rather than the outcome. Teach kids that trying hard matters. (Think Tortoise versus Hare.)

"Hard work trumps talent every time."

—Vinky, father of three

At a pool party, kids were having a diving contest and pretending they were in the Olympics. The parents were judging. A kid did a belly flop. "Eight and a half!" one mom yelled. Ouch. Really? Clearly, the parents were being very generous with their calls. Every child seemed to earn an eight, nine, or ten.

One bold mom saw her kid dive and said, "Your feet were not touching. I will give you a five." The other parents looked horrified and wondered if the kid would storm off the board and cry. But he didn't. He returned to the board looking more determined and continued to practice the dive for the next hour, getting better each time.

The other kids had stopped diving after receiving their nines and tens. This kid, on the other hand, came home with a goody bag full of lessons, such as "The harder you work, the more you will improve." He discovered that he could trust his mom to tell him the truth. She didn't treat him as if he were fragile, or prop him up with overblown compliments. She had faith that he was strong enough to learn from honest feedback. And so he did.

"Parents today think that everyone needs a ribbon, and that everyone should get a trophy. Parents today are so afraid of the psychological consequences of disappointing their kid that they forget to think of the psychological consequences of not being disappointed."

—Eric Wlasak, elementary school teacher

Let's stop heaping on the false praise and let kids dive into life knowing the real score.

Toolbox for Building Resilient Kids

- When in doubt, stay out. Allow them to feel and experience their own accomplishment without jumping in. Let it be theirs.
- Let them struggle. Allow them to fumble with a task until they get it themselves.
- Check in. Is what you're fixing about your emotional need or theirs?
- Ask questions rather than offering solutions. Help them problem solve rather than solve their problems.
- Let them get emotionally frustrated. Allow them to learn to self-soothe.
- Teach the perspective that failure is not final.
- Teach them 100 percent accountability for their choices.
- Give specific, authentic praise that feels genuine. Praise effort, not outcome.
- Keep in mind: "It is easier to build strong children than to repair broken men."—Frederick Douglass

Shrink Notes

Look, No Hands!

1. The packaging instructions for childhood should read "Handle with care," not "Fragile, will break."
2. Don't bubble wrap the kid *or* the road.
3. Our job is not to prevent our kids from failing; it is to teach them that failure is part of the process of success.
4. Get comfortable being uncomfortable.
5. Don't be a human pacifier. Let your kids learn to soothe themselves.
6. Dependency breeds resentment.
7. Make sure kids do chores and have summer jobs to learn responsibility and accountability.
8. False praise is just that. Take the *-est* out of your compliments.
9. Allow children to practice being disappointed.
10. Ideally, parents work themselves out of a job.

CHAPTER FOUR

Being an Emotional Grown-up

> My children are the most enriching personal development seminar that I have ever taken.
>
> —Bianca, Waldorf teacher

When I was a medical student, a dad brought his ten-year-old boy into the emergency room after he'd fallen hard during their father-son camping trip.

"I feel so bad," the dad began. "I travel a lot for work and I really wanted to spend these four days alone with my son in nature, bonding with him." While they were hiking, the boy fell and gashed his knee. The father continued the story as I cleaned the boy's wound. "In spite of the fall, we had an amazing trip, and I have never felt closer to him."

Another doctor came in to suture the wound. He carried a large needle full of lidocaine. Reading the fear on his son's face, this lovely father rubbed the boy's back and said, "I am here, son, I am right here."

The minute the needle pierced the boy's skin, he cried out: "I want MOMMY!"

Ouch, poor Dad.

"I know how badly you want Mommy to be here with you. I wish she could be here with you right now."

How impressive. The dad set aside his own need to be needed and validated his son's feelings. The accident might have left the kid with a scar on his knee, but this kind of parenting will prevent scars from forming on his heart.

Being emotionally grown-up often requires setting aside your own needs so you can be in service to your child.

The more self-aware we are, the better we can parent. Our parenting is directly related to our own self-understanding. Parenting is an opportunity to parent yourself, so that you can parent your child.

DON'T INVERT THE ROLES

Years ago, I was scheduled to see a six-year-old boy who was about to be thrown out of his second Chicago school. I tried to imagine what a six-year-old could have done to get himself into so much trouble at such a young age.

I did not have to wait long to find out. The answer came flying through my office door. Derek exploded into the room. He began exploring my office by yanking books off the shelves and onto the floor. After jumping on my couch, he headed over to my desk. I glanced at his mother and grandmother to gauge their reaction to all this mayhem. They were unfazed.

"Please sit down, Derek," I began.

After introducing myself to his family, I asked Derek to

tell me about himself. He immediately jumped up and stood on my couch, put his hands on his hips with a swagger, and boomed: "This is my mom and grandma. I have no dad and I am the MAN of the house."

I have to admit, it was quite a spectacle. I peered over to his mom, who was smiling proudly. Then I looked back at Derek and said, "Derek, you are no man. You are a six-year-old little boy."

In an instant, all the big-boy bravado faded and he quietly shrunk down into the couch, deflated—but simultaneously relieved.

No child should ever be "the man of the house." Parents need to be emotional grown-ups so that kids can get to be kids. It is way too burdensome for a child to have to be the grown-up. They don't have the skills. They can't even reach the sink or tie their shoes. They're too young to take care of themselves, much less to take care of you.

But kids are highly intuitive, and when the wounds of their parents become visible, children will try to rescue their parents. A child unconsciously thinks, Let me care for her, so that maybe she will get around to caring for me. A child feels responsible for shoring up a parent's emotional well-being. Or, in Derek's case, filling a vacant role. This is the stuff that prevents children from fully depending on their parents. They don't get to be children who rely on a strong, safe mom or dad. If you skip that phase, the road to real emotional independence is blocked. Dependency must come first. Derek needs to be a boy before he can be a real man.

One divorced woman at an outpatient clinic told me, "When I come home from work, my son [age five] rubs my feet and pours me lemonade. Isn't that sweet?"

Shrink says: not so much.

Your child is not your friend, your masseuse, or your confidant. You could almost see that boy asking, "How was your day, honey? Would you like me to draw you a bath?" He so strongly felt his mother's need to be cared for that he stepped up and did it. But he is just a little fella, and his shoulders can't really support her weight. When children take on the caregiving role, they never just relax and get taken care of themselves. The roles get inverted. That puts them on guard and builds up their defenses. If they do not have nurturing parents, they cannot let themselves be vulnerable, and the loss of vulnerability is a loss of our true selves. This is how kids start to grow heart armor.

But wait, you might think, it's reciprocal—the mom also comforts the child when he needs her. That's probably true. But relationships at a child's early stage of development should not be reciprocal. Parenting is not "I'll rub your feet, you rub mine." When ducklings imprint, they follow their mom around. Mama ducks don't follow back.

> *"Being a parent is not transactional. We don't get what we give. It is the ultimate pay-it-forward endeavor: we are good parents not so they will be loving enough to stay with us, but so they will be strong enough to leave us."*
>
> —Anna Quindlen, *Lots of Candles, Plenty of Cake*

In order for our children to grow independent, first they must be allowed into emotional dependency. If they acutely feel your need, they will not have that opportunity. The roles will become reversed. Kids are perceptive. If they see their parent in need, they will play the role of caregiver.

But this comes at a great price. When a parent's needs reign supreme, they take up all the air in the room. The child might seem like a little adult, but internally his development gets stunted while he is emotionally tending to his parents. He's so aware of their needs that he has to swallow his own.

If a child continually swallows his own needs, he will grow further and further away from his own vulnerability and authentic self. When you get away from your true self, you lose access to your full range of emotions and start erecting a false self that protects you from more pain. This is the opposite of self-esteem. This is my bread and butter as a psychiatrist, excavating the true self that was buried—buried to survive childhood.

"All children have a deep need to be loved. If they perceive that a parent is fragile, a child will learn to parent their parent. Kids learn early that they need to go through the side door to get their needs met. Many of my clients retell stories of cleaning up the house to try to make their moms happy. But only parents can fix themselves. The child is powerless."

—Marcy Cole, PsyD

EVOLVE BEYOND YOUR PRIMITIVE EMOTIONS

Being a parent does not make you an emotional grown-up any more than standing in the White House makes you the president.

Many adults act like children because they missed having

their dependency needs met, and therefore these needs keep returning in adulthood. Think about the date who never asks about you (because he was never truly made central), the guy who flips the finger on the highway (because his parents never helped him regulate his emotions), or the spouse who needs constant reassurance (because she missed out on having a secure attachment to her parents).

I am oversimplifying here, but don't miss the message: kids desperately need their parents to be the grown-ups.

So if your child is having a meltdown in public, don't react by saying you're going to leave him or her in the airport or grocery store. (A) It's childish. (B) You don't mean it. (C) Empty threats erode trust. (D) You're trying to control through intimidation. Not a winning strategy.

Old-school parenting was based on threats, yelling, hitting, and withdrawal of love. Trying to shape behavior with primitive and childlike antics is not a grown-up game plan. It just leaves children lonely and scared.

> *"It is better to bind your children to you by a feeling of respect and by gentleness than by fear."*
>
> —Terence, ancient Roman dramatist

Children who are scared of their parents are truly powerless. Having an unsafe, emotionally volatile parent is the quickest route to a buried self. Having an unpredictable parent whom you can only intermittently rely on prevents a secure and safe attachment. Kids have to depend on their parents for food, clothing, shelter, and protection from physical and emotional harm.

Children who are physically or emotionally mistreated by their parents are in a terrible bind. Children still need to rely on their parents but simultaneously fear them.

I witnessed a devastating example of this while working one night in the emergency room.

A four-year-old girl was brought in with severe water burns from having been put in a scalding bath as a punishment for misbehavior. It was soul crushing to watch her in excruciating pain as the mom confessed to the crime. I called the police and the Department of Children and Family Services. There was almost a moment of relief, then shock returned. The little girl began wailing, "Mommy, Mommy," and grasping for her mother as the police took her away. No matter how much pain her mother had caused, her mother was still the person she wanted.

We all crave the love of our mother, however flawed she may be.

I am sorry to even share this story, but it shows so clearly the unthinkable dilemma that kids face when parents can't control their rage.

Thankfully, most examples are not that extreme—and if you care enough to read this book, abuse probably isn't in your repertoire. But, of course, we all have days when we lose it, and we want to minimize that damage. If you are the protector but simultaneously the source of fear, your child will never be able to truly rely on you.

"Sometimes my mom was a mom, sometimes a monster. I guess I was raised by a momster."

—Tales from the couch

Parents are supposed to be slaying the metaphorical monsters, not embodying them. When you are emotionally out of control and your house is filled with chaos, kids learn to tread lightly so as not to ignite minefields. When the minefields explode, fear fills your child, which sets off a cascade of toxic neurochemical changes starting with an elevated level of cortisol, triggering a fight-or-flight arousal. This puts your child's brain in survival mode instead of growth mode and interferes with the development of a resilient brain.

If you feel your control or patience waning, remind yourself of the role you want to be remembered for: hero, not villain; protector, not persecutor.

To be that heroic, you have to get your own stuff out of the way first. You have to raise yourself so that you can raise your child. You might have to glance back to find the underdeveloped pieces of yourself. Nobody prepares us for this part of parenting, but it is essential for success.

THE GHOSTS OF PARENTS PAST

It's hard to give what you never got. It is a great advantage to have come from great parents. If you did not have that advantage, let's face it, your job is tougher. Being a parent might bring back painful memories that you thought you had pocketed away.

But darkness is an opportunity for light. In order to find that light, you might need to face the ghosts of parents past.

Look at how Ebenezer Scrooge, the lonely and unhappy man in Dickens's *A Christmas Carol*, found salvation in facing his childhood ghosts. He had to examine the pain of his youth to reawaken as a happy, changed man in the present.

If we do not glance back and gain insight into our own childhood story, we might automatically repeat the same mistakes with our children. Our mission is to add conscious intent to our parenting so our history does not become our child's destiny. We have to work actively so we don't default to the way we were parented.

You wouldn't cough on your child without covering your mouth. So make sure your unresolved issues don't infect your children.

"My parents' flaws and weaknesses became the fuel for my own development."

—Seattle mom

Looking back on your childhood wounds can be very painful. But when you can see clearly what you missed as a child, you can mourn that loss and then realize you have the power to re-parent yourself. What do I wish I would have heard as a child? What do I wish I would have received? How do I wish I would have been loved?

Give yourself the unconditional love that you always craved from your parents. Love yourself enough to let go of the toxic comments that you know, deep in your heart, do not apply to you. Extricate them from your sense of self. Be the kind of parent—first to yourself and then to your kids—that you always wanted. That is how you rid your ghosts of their haunting power.

A mom in my parenting group told a story about her four-year-old daughter, Darcy, who would go to bed at night sucking her thumb and cuddling her blanket. One night, Darcy's grandparents were reading her a bedtime story. The scene touched Darcy's mom, Janet, until Janet heard her mother shame her daughter in an effort to help her "grow up."

"You are too old for blankies, Darcy. Blankies are for babies. You are a big girl. You don't need that blanket," Grandma declared.

Janet saw the shame on her daughter's face, which brought her back to the way that she had been shamed as a child. She remembered how her need to be dependent had always made her mom uncomfortable. Now in the role of parent, Janet was not going to let history repeat itself. She intervened.

"Mom, Darcy loves her blanket. She will know when she's ready to let it go."

Darcy looked soothed, and Janet felt empowered. Janet met her daughter where *she* was, not where Grandma wanted her to be. Janet had protected her child in a way that she had not been able to protect her younger self. With age and wisdom, Grandma saw her mistake and apologized to her daughter and granddaughter. It was very reparative for all of them.

A few months later Janet went to check on a sleeping Darcy and spied the blanket at the end of the bed. The next night she found it in the closet—where it still remains.

Undoing the programming of your parents is not easy, so get help if you need it. If you do the tough work of facing those ghosts of parents past, you can liberate yourself from the legacy of parenting patterns that no longer serve you. Keep what you loved and discard the rest. You are the parent now. You have the power to make that change.

RUPTURE AND REPAIR

"Never ruin an apology with an excuse."

—Benjamin Franklin

At a mommy-and-me group with newborns, I overheard a mom say to her baby, "I am so sorry, honey, I forgot to bring your diaper bag, and you need to be changed. I am new at this, and I hope you will be patient with me as we learn together."

One of the other moms overheard, rolled her eyes, and said, "I would not worry about it. First off, she does not understand you, and, second of all, she will not remember this."

The other mom smiled. "I know. But I am going to mess up, and I just want to get in the habit of apologizing to my child, and cut myself some slack as well."

No parent always gets it right the first time. Or the second or third. Parenting is the ultimate in on-the-job training. You'll forget to bring a diaper bag, lose your temper, say the wrong things, let frustration throw off your delivery. You'll get harried. You will judge with your head instead of listening with your heart.

Go easy on yourself. Parenting is a dynamic process under the most stressful, always-juggling, short-on-time, short-on-sleep conditions. We are human, and this is a very human job with a high degree of human error. Lucky for us, kids are forgiving. And human error creates a wonderful opportunity for real closeness. When there is rupture, follow it with repair. Medicate the situation with your apology. Own your mistake. It is very disarming. It is also a very attractive thing to teach your kids.

"My greatest strength as a mother was my ability to self-reflect. I always admitted to my kids when I made a mistake. I gave heartfelt apologies. I talked about how I would do it differently the next time. I let them in on my thought process. I showed compassion for them as well as for myself."

—Mom of two

"Parents today are so hung up on being perfect. (By the way, there is no such thing.) Just be aware and address your mistakes openly with your child. It models something for them, something they could not get if you were perfect."

—Julie Gedden, MD, psychiatrist

Good parents evolve right alongside their children. What a gift it is to know that when we mess up we can circle back and make amends. Apology will not undermine your authority. It actually strengthens your credibility as a trustworthy leader.

The beauty of parenting is that there is no statute of limitations on repair.

"As I aged and evolved, my parenting got better. But I still felt bad about some mistakes that I made when my sons were little," one father said.

Before his twins went off to college, he took them on a weekend river-rafting trip.

"My goal for the trip was to celebrate my sons, but also to make peace. I made a playbook in my head of my parenting highlights and low moments. We floated down the river, and I was surprised, but I got really emotional. I cried telling them how bad I felt about their childhood. I had messed up. I explained that I had real financial strain at the time, which I let interfere with my parenting, and that that was a mistake. In the early years, I was sort of sleepwalking through parenting, but now I have woken up. If I could go back and do it again, I would do it entirely differently, and I am deeply sorry. I apologized for yelling so much, being too harsh with my punishments, and not spending enough time with them. I told them that they, along with their mom, were the most important people in my whole world, and that I never had meant to hurt them. The three of us hugged each other and cried as we drifted down the river."

Apologies and changed behavior are healing at every age.

In the last few years, my colleagues and I have noticed a trend of parents making appointments with their adult children. For whatever reason, their relationships had become strained, and they wanted to find a way back to closeness. Before my therapy sessions, I encourage parents to put aside their defensiveness, to truly hear their children, to not make excuses, and to sincerely apologize for past mistakes. Empathy opens the door to vulnerability. Use it to create greater intimacy.

Again, self-awareness and willingness to change are necessary for healing.

One grandmother felt bad when her grown children constantly reminded her of how quick-tempered she had been with them. The adult kids braced themselves whenever a grandchild broke or spilled something. But Grandma had decided to do it differently this time around. "No big deal" became her grandmotherly motto. When her grandson threw up on her expensive rug, everyone anticipated an explosion. But she had grown beyond her old ways. Instead she reassured the sick boy. "This rug isn't as important as you. I don't care about the rug, I care about you."

Her kids were astonished by the turnaround. But they were also comforted to know that the opportunity for repair and transformational healing never ends.

CHECK YOUR EGO

It's really hard to get your ego and judgment out of parenting. But that, too, is part of being a grown-up. The trick is identifying it so that you can best manage it.

Setting your stuff aside clears the way for you to see your children for who they truly are.

One beautiful fall day, parents and kids took up tug-of-war at a preschool. After a lot of back and forth, the parents gave one final staged pull and let the kids win.

The five-year-olds cheered and jumped up and down with excitement. Except for Greg, who ran up to his mom with tears pouring down his face. Greg's mom could not figure out why her child was the only one sobbing after winning tug-of-war and grew uncomfortable at the glances and comments from other moms. She started to grill her son: "Why are you crying? Nobody else is crying. You are embarrassing me."

Then she caught herself and traded criticism for understanding. She took a few breaths and knelt down next to her son and wiped away his tears. She gentled her tone. "Tell me what's going on."

A sobbing Greg explained his confusion. "We didn't

really win, Mom, did we? How could we? We are half your size. Do my friends really believe we won?"

"You are right, sweetheart," Greg's mom soothed, "you did not really win."

"Then I feel really alone," Greg said.

Greg's mom went immediately from embarrassment to empathy. The real tug-of-war is often the parent's internal struggle, wrestling our own ego to the ground so that we can see our children for who they are—different and special. If we let go of the rope of our preconceptions, our children's true, beautiful selves shine through.

Let's replay what Greg's mom did right.

- She caught herself being judgmental and trying to silence her child.
- She self-corrected and knelt down to meet her kid where *he* was.
- She was on her kid's side of the lesson.
- She truly heard, understood, and saw her child.
- She deepened trust, proving to her child that it was safe to come to her when he was hurting.

"When it comes to parenting, check your ego at the door."

—Longtime teacher

It is hard for any parent to set aside his or her own emotions. It's even tougher if you have narcissistic tendencies. Parents are supposed to mirror and reflect their children's feelings and experiences. That is how children begin to understand themselves and form their own identities. Attuned parents see their children for who they are. Narcissistic parents are blinded by their own needs, which overshadow the needs and emotions of their children. It's hard to grow healthy kids in shadows.

Narcissists' profound need for attention, praise, and reassurance subverts everyone else's needs. They have a way of making everything about them, taking everything personally. "How could you do this to me?" is a common refrain. They are easily offended, and, when injured, they are prone to lose their temper.

The whole family often caters to the narcissists. Their children learn to tiptoe around their fiery emotions. Picking up on their parent's vulnerability, intuitive children try to shore up their parent. And thus the mirror is reversed. The child has to mirror the parent instead of the parent mirroring the child.

Children of such parents are so busy tending their parents' emotional well-being that they lose touch with their own needs. And on those rare occasions when their own needs make themselves known, children are forced to choose between their happiness and their parents'. Most often their own needs are sacrificed to keep peace in the family. They learn that they will receive love not by being themselves, but by pleasing others.

Lily was trying on prom dresses in a department store dressing room. The store was getting ready to close, and Lily was acutely aware of her mom's desire to buy a dress and leave. Mom's need to be done dampened Lily's excitement about finding a dress she felt good in for this special rite of passage.

Her mother said, "I found the perfect dress for you!" and

held up an ugly dress with red and white stripes. Lily took one look and immediately hated it. Masking her disappointment, she put it on anyway.

"It's perfect, I love it!" Mom said, not even seeing how unhappy Lily was. Now the girl was in a troublesome bind. Which mirror should she attend to—the literal one, which clearly showed a dress she would be embarrassed to wear, or the mirror she was used to reflecting and pleasing?

The daughter tentatively expressed her discomfort. Her mom's agitation flared. Lily reflexively changed her tune: "I guess you're right, it does fit well," she said, flatly. Her mom smiled, feeling much better. And for just that moment, Lily felt better, too. But not really.

On prom night, Lily walked self-consciously down the stairs to greet her date. His disappointed first words—"Red stripes?"—were crushing.

Long after the prom dress was discarded, the memory of catering to her mom's needs on her special night—and many other nights—lingered. Twenty years later, she asked in therapy why she didn't trust her own instincts, why she had trouble saying no and expressing her true feelings.

Lily finally realized: "I was so busy keeping my mom afloat, I wasn't sure where my mom ended and I began. I never really had a voice as a kid."

This is why children of narcissists often show up in therapy as adults; they are trying to find—and free—their authentic selves. Surviving childhood meant catering to their parents and subverting themselves. They worry that if they assert themselves in their current relationships, they will risk losing love. Or they grow up to have narcissistic traits themselves. Neither scenario is optimal. But if you were parented by a narcissist, the legacy can end with you.

How can you do better? First, check in with yourself when you feel agitated. Ask yourself: "Am I recognizing what my kid is feeling or am I too caught up in my own emotions?" Slow down for just a moment. Give yourself time to reflect. Understand what is activating you so you can offer constructive guidance instead of reacting with anger or by withdrawing love.

Remember that your children are not an extension of you. Sameness is not closeness. They are their own people, and their feelings and behavior don't have to be the same as yours. I never loved the term *Mini-Me*. Because if you are you and they are you, then there's no room for them to be them.

Sadly, narcissism is often multigenerational. Parents who never had their needs met are incapable of meeting those of their children—unless they are willing to step up and be the cycle breakers.

CHECK YOUR EMOTIONS

One spring morning I was sitting on a bench at a preschool chatting with Kevin, a wonderful dad. We were having a lovely talk when his daughter Patty ran up to him in tears.

"Jenna said that she does not want to play with me anymore," she sobbed in a deep, staccato cry that tugged at my heartstrings.

"I bet that does not feel good," he gently validated. He gave her a long cuddle and wiped away her tears. "What are you going to do now?" he asked, throwing the resiliency ball back in her court.

"Well, I guess I can play with a girl I know with brown eyes and brown hair."

"You mean *you*?" the dad asked warmly.

"Yes," Patty said with a smile.

"Great idea," Kevin replied, and off she skipped.

"Wow, that was such a beautiful intervention," I said. "That was textbook great parenting."

He looked at me and said, "That little Jenna is a bitch!"

I nearly fell off the bench laughing. I was so surprised by his real feelings. He was just as upset as Patty was, but he knew his frustration wouldn't help her. So he set aside his emotions so that he could give her the calm guidance she needed. And he did such a good job that I did not even know his true feelings.

Being an emotional grown-up does not mean that you don't have your own feelings or that you are not stirred by your child's pain, but that you don't further complicate things by piling your feelings onto theirs.

"When my kid goes down the rabbit hole, I try so hard not to go down with him. But it's tough not to go tumbling down after him."

—Mother of three

By staying out of the rabbit hole, Patty's dad was able to act as an emotional holding tank for his daughter's intense feelings.

One of your big jobs as parents is to be an emotion coach. You need to teach kids to regulate their big feelings, not project your feelings onto them. Because we care, our emotions often escalate right alongside our children's. When they are upset, we may match their emotion and pile our upset feelings onto theirs. Keep the focus on them and their feelings. Then make separate time for yours.

SELF-CARE

Why is it that we pay more attention to recharging our smartphones than to recharging ourselves? If we were smart, we'd pay attention when our battery light started flashing "low." Refresh yourself so you can parent with new power.

I'm not going to tell you how to reboot—you know whether a walk, a talk with friends, music, meditation, a good workout, or something else will renew your spirit. But I will say that you should make the time to do it.

Self-care is not selfish. It is essential. Nothing interferes more with parenting than stress. Financial, social, medical, work-related pressures all drain you. Kids pick up on your energy, good or bad. That's why it's so crucial to take time for you.

One husband worried that his wife was taking time for an affair when suspicious charges showed up on her credit card. Immediately recognizing credit card fraud, the wife laughed at the preposterous notion that she had the energy to be duplicitous.

"I can't even imagine having an affair," the wife exclaimed. "First of all, who has time? Second of all, my children are hanging on me all day long, demanding things of me, calling my name. I don't want one more person needing anything from me—let alone touching me. My idea of an affair would be to check into a hotel room by myself with a stack of books and a remote control and absolutely *nobody* even knowing I was there. Don't get me wrong, I love my husband and my kids. But a night alone? Now, that would be an affair!"

Parents often feel overwhelmed. But some days are worse—especially for women at certain times of the month.

PMS—and its more severe form, premenstrual dysphoric disorder—can make moms feel not like themselves. I cannot even count the number of women I hear in my office report, "I feel like Jekyll and Hyde." This is not sexist; it is biology. The highest rate of psychiatric hospital admissions for women occurs between menses and menopause. The highest incidence of depression and anxiety occurs during the reproductive years. So hormonal fluctuations make us most vulnerable at the very time we're striving to be good parents. Don't discount that.

Being an emotional grown-up means knowing when you are spent. Moms and dads, don't just ignore your stress, because it will come out as impatience and irritability, which we struggle with enough as parents. Make time to relax and recharge your battery in whatever way works for you.

Every morning the life coach James Rouse meditates, eats a nutritious breakfast, and works out in nature. All this before he flips pancakes for his daughters, writes his books, teaches his seminars, and helps people live healthier lives. Where in the world does he find the time?

"It is not something you *find*, it's something you *create*," Rouse said.

For some people, that ideal feels out of reach. That's when you get creative.

Pam was at her wit's end when her kids were little and her husband was gone for work. She had no money, no sitter, and no way to walk out the door. So she grabbed a diary she had written on a trip to Europe after college and got lost in it.

"I was deep into it when my kids came in arguing about something and wanting me to resolve it for them," Pam said. "I remember looking up at them and saying, 'I am not here. I am on a boat sailing to England and I am having a marvelous time!' They shook their heads and looked at each other, as if to say 'She's loonier than we thought.' Then they went back to playing, fight forgotten."

A refreshed parent is more likely to be a good parent. So take a few minutes to sail off in solitude, even if it is only in your mind.

USE YOUR LIFELINES

Sometimes when our kids are struggling, we get stuck. We feel like Sisyphus, trying to roll the boulder uphill only to watch it roll down again. It's awful when you try every solution you can think of, yet nothing seems to work. Welcome to parenting.

Don't try this alone. Use your lifelines. Get help. Phone a friend. Ask an expert. Visit your child's teachers. Talk to your pediatrician. Call a therapist. Get a book and look for ideas. Ask a great parent, your minister, a rabbi, or your kid's coach. Just reach out. When we are stuck, an objective opinion is invaluable. Collaboration always helps. Create your own parenting Rolodex so you can have the support you need.

It's so reassuring to learn that other people have struggled with the same things—and found their way out. Getting another perspective can make you feel like you are not alone, and it might give you a parenting pearl that will make a difference for you and your child.

Parenting has so many roles: chef, chauffeur, keeper of the calendar, personal shopper, personal hygienist, nail clipper, nose wiper, manners police, nurse, emotion coach, mentor, role model, visionary, and soul guide. Who could possibly do it alone?

"My mom went through a very challenging time when she was raising us, but instead of falling apart, she got help. She went out looking for solutions, and she found them. Her example has empowered me to do the same."

—Loren, mother of two

Emotional grown-ups ask for help and guidance. Don't make it a one-person show. Build your own supporting cast. Use your lifelines to help shape a little life.

NAVIGATING ROUGH WATERS

"Good families—even great families—are off track 90 percent of the time! The key is that they have a sense of the destination. The hope lies in the vision and in the plan and in the courage to keep coming back time and time again."

—Stephen Covey, *The 7 Habits of Highly Effective Families*

Parenthood is a courageous journey. I guarantee you will hit some rough seas as captain. Seas so rough that you lose your balance, feel sick to your stomach, and even lose sight of land. Kids blow off course. They have setbacks and need to begin again. We have to be our kids' North Star.

Development is never a straight line. My patients who have worked through enormous challenges, like losing hundreds of pounds or staying sober, all share a windy road to success. Often the turning point was in how kindly they spoke to themselves when they veered off course. Treating themselves with compassion and appreciating a partial victory got them back on track. In shaping behavior, give full credit for partial success. Know that kids will grow past the dips and swells of growing up. I once heard a doctor say, "Don't worry, no girl walks down the aisle with a pacifier in her mouth."

But that perspective can be hard to keep. We love our kids so deeply that we worry that any rough waters they face will never calm again. Perspective will help you both find safe harbor.

When I worked in inpatient psychiatry, I witnessed some very dark storms. I tried to hold a loving space for people during extremely difficult times. One night, a mother brought in her twenty-three-year-old daughter, who was having her first manic episode with psychotic features. She thought that her phone was being bugged and that all of her law school professors were really spies.

Her mother's devastation was palpable. Her daughter was diagnosed with bipolar disorder and started on lithium. The mother would visit her daily in a locked-down psychiatric unit. Her mother cried to me one night, saying that all of her daughter's dreams of becoming a lawyer and a wife and a mother were now dashed.

Though her daughter would have bipolar disorder for life, I told the mother that once her daughter was stabilized, if she continued to take her medications, she would be able to return to law school. We discussed how many well-known and high-functioning people shared her daughter's diagnosis. She clung to her rosary beads as we talked. She said that she would keep building a bridge in her mind to that image. We held a space of hope.

A few years later, the mother wrote me saying that her daughter had graduated from law school and that she was engaged. How far we had come from that night when she gripped her rosary beads.

No matter what difficulties you run into with your children, keep imagining them at their best. Believing things will get better gives you both something to hold on to until they do.

Therapy Tools That Work for Parenting

- See the blossom while looking at the bud.
- Visualize your child's greatest self; hold that image in difficult times.
- Listen to understand, not to judge.
- Hold a loving space for negative or charged emotions.
- Create a safe place for feeling known and understood.
- Pay attention to the emotion behind the words.
- Own and apologize for your mistakes.
- Circle back if you miss something.

Things Therapists Often Hear

- "My parents withdrew love. When I disappointed them, they would give me the silent treatment."

- "They shamed me when I misbehaved. I still hear their criticism in my head."
- "Their emotional volatility made me feel unsafe."
- "My parents' needs overshadowed mine. My parents' needs reigned supreme."
- "My parents acted like children. They would yell and pout if they did not get their way."
- "If I disagreed with my parents, they freaked out and took it personally."
- "Feeling close to my parents meant taking care of them and swallowing me."

Things Therapists Rarely Hear

- "My parents loved me unconditionally."
- "My parents set clear and consistent limits."
- "My parents taught me values and often said no."
- "My parents took care of their emotional needs so that they could attend to mine."
- "My parents owned their mistakes and learned from them."
- "My parents were a safe haven. I could come to them with everything."
- "My parents showed me the type of person I want to be."

Shrink Notes

Being an Emotional Grown-up

1. Address the ghosts of your own parents so they don't continue to haunt you.
2. Get your ego out of the game. Ask: Is this about me or my kid?
3. Own your mistakes. Follow rupture with repair.
4. Use your lifelines. Phone a friend, ask an expert, get the support you need.
5. Self-care is not selfish; it is essential.
6. Visualize the bridge to the future. Hold the perspective.
7. Don't invert the roles.
8. Get out of the way; don't pile your feelings on top of theirs.
9. Grab hold of your emotions; be a consistent parent, not a volatile parent.
10. Grow yourself so you can grow your child.

CHAPTER FIVE

Trash the Trash Talk

Whoever said "Sticks and stones may break my bones, but names will never hurt me" was completely wrong. We all skinned our knees as kids. Those wounds are long forgotten. . . . Angry outbursts, insults we remember forever. . . . Words wound in deep and powerful ways.

—Rabbi Steven Leder, in a Yom Kippur sermon, 2011

While I was studying for my medical school entrance exams, I taught as a substitute in a midwestern elementary school. One day an announcement on the loudspeaker told the children that, due to extreme cold weather, recess would be indoors. Immediately I heard a little girl wrangle a boy into playing house. "I will be the mommy, and you be the daddy," she said.

Just when I was thinking how adorable kindergartners are, the little girl moved right up to the boy's face, pointed her finger at him, and snapped, "I am so sick and tired of your golf trips, and no more gin and tonics!"

Like so many men who look blankly at their wives, the boy realized that this game of house was not so fun, so he shrugged his shoulders and walked away.

This is the ultimate cautionary tale in watching what you model.

As I've said, the language you use in your home—whether directed at your partner, your kids, or yourself—becomes the soundtrack in your children's head. Children learn from what they see and hear. So go easy on the trash talk.

I'm not talking about the sharp elbows and rough language of the NBA. I'm talking about the everyday conversation in our homes. Often we don't even hear ourselves being critical, shameful, or harsh. We think we're being instructive. But we need to start listening to our words and gentling our tone so we don't thoughtlessly dump negativity onto the people we love the most.

Trash talking can be extremely subtle and even seem benign. In family parenting sessions, parents are often shocked at the things that hurt their children's feelings. What you think is just observational may sound charged or pointed to your children. We must practice choosing our words with grace.

Otherwise our children—along with our spouses and ourselves—will bear the brunt of our careless words. Think back to dating. The loving gazes, the playful tone, the charm. You spoke with affection and love. Let's add some of that care back into our families. Let's treat them like the people they are—our nearest and dearest.

"Our children are our guests for eighteen years. We have to treat our guests with the utmost respect."

—Jackie, mom of three

NO TRASH TALKING YOUR SPOUSE OR YOUR EX

"I don't think anything is lost on children. Kids absorb all of the family dynamics. They are witnessed and marked, as if they are breathing these relationships."

—Ben, father

How you and your partner or ex treat each other is an integral part of your parenting. Even in a strained relationship, how you talk to each other and how you resolve conflict teaches your children about love and respect. What you model becomes the template for your children's behavior. It provides the foundation of your home. It gives them safety or creates instability.

"As a kid, I had a recurring dream that I was walking on creaky floors. One night I dreamed that I stepped on a floorboard, and it broke, and I fell underneath my house, and my whole house came tumbling down on top of me."

—Tales from the couch

You don't need to be a psychiatrist to analyze that. This child had been exposed to so much marital battling that there was no peace in his home, or respite in his dreams.

A loving relationship creates safety for your children. But if you are struggling with a difficult marriage or divorce, it is so hard to take the high road. You feel angry, hurt, and emotionally spent. It's extremely challenging to protect your kids from your feelings.

"I don't think that people who have not been through a divorce can even understand how devastating it is. You wake up one morning without your kids and you feel as if your limbs have been ripped off, and then you still have to deal with your ex."

—Divorced mother

"I was married for seventeen years. I have four children and a very demanding career. One day my wife told me that she was leaving me for another man. I felt blindsided. In one moment, it felt like everything I loved was gone. After great sadness came great anger. I made a very conscious effort to shield my kids from all of that."

—Divorced father

When you are in the raw stages of pain, keeping your feelings from your kids is exceedingly difficult. But I beg you to try. Kids feel the body blows of parental conflict. As one young man explained, "When my mom would trash talk my dad, it was as if she was trash talking half of my DNA!"

Words and feelings matter. Spoken or not.

"My mom never actually said anything bad about my dad. She did not have to. Her eye rolling and the tone she used when she talked about him spoke loudly enough."

—College student

Verbal or nonverbal, when you trash talk your ex, you are trash talking your kid by proxy!

Kids have bionic eyes and ears. They see and hear it all. Even if you think you are being subtle, you are not. It is not going over your child's head. Do not vent, eye roll, or trash talk your ex or partner when your child is home. Make your house a sanctuary, not a battlefield.

Unfortunately, some homes are battlefields of physical and emotional abuse. That's not what I'm talking about here. In those situations, you have to get children to safety and let them know that the adult behavior is unacceptable—and that they did nothing to deserve it. In such cases, everyone will need professional help.

What I'm talking about are the charged feelings that come when relationships fall apart, when marriage is a struggle, or when day-to-day frustrations interfere with caring communication.

When you're talking about your child's other parent, try to imagine you're talking directly to your child. Try to think how your child will hear it and feel it. That should give you pause. Honesty and directness don't have to sting. They can still be presented in a loving manner.

I know that thinking before you speak and gentling your language can be tough, but what you say and how you behave have far-reaching psychological implications.

"It was very hard for me to be honorable about my ex-husband. I bad-mouthed him, and that was a huge mistake. I am a grandmother now, and I realize how my anger toward my ex still affects my grown children to this day. My biggest regret is that I did not shield them from that."

—Micki, grandma

Whenever you can, protect kids from your charged feelings. Children need to believe in both parents, trust them, and adore them. Children often idealize their parents—at least until adolescence. The teenage years are typically when kids begin to realize that their parents are flawed—lovable but human—and Mom and Dad gradually fall from grace.

The key word here is *gradual*. We want to step down from the pedestal gently, even gracefully, if possible. It leaves our children with less psychological bruising. To protect them, we want to protect our spouse or ex from falling off too soon—even when our more primitive instincts want to give him a big old shove. We do not need to push our coparents into the gutter by pointing out all their flaws, modeling contempt, or having a partnership imbued with constant conflict.

Just realize that your children know what you mean when you say "I am not going to say anything bad about your mom BUT . . ." or "You are just like your dad." They know this is not a compliment. The high road is harder to climb, but everyone is so much healthier when you aim for the top.

"It is parental conflict—not divorce itself—that places children at risk in virtually every area in their lives. In fact, children from intact families with high conflict fare no better in standardized psychological tests than those whose parents are divorced. Conversely, most children of divorce who witness little conflict between their parents do as well as children from intact homes."

—M. Gary Neuman, *Helping Your Kids Cope with Divorce the Sandcastles Way*

When a mother or father trash talks their spouse or ex, the child is forced to defend the other parent. Try not to let home feel like a competition in which a child has to pick sides. Don't discuss your relationship woes with your kids. Remember that our biggest task as parents is to build secure attachments, not competing ones. You don't need to be the special or favorite parent. Two secure attachments, if possible, are better than one. You want your child to feel safe and loved by both of you.

"As a teacher you know right away which divorced families are still a team and working together. They use the words we *and* our child *and* our family. *It is clear that they coparent from separate homes. They put their issues aside for the sake of the child. On the opposite end, I have parents sit at the same small table at conferences, with their arms crossed. Exasperated, they look at me and say, 'Tell his father to get him to bed earlier' and 'Tell his mother that she needs to make sure he does his homework.' I think, You tell him, he is right there."*

—Elementary school teacher

"Parents want to do the right thing. They love their kids; they just can't separate their personal feelings and problems from their parenting. They should. Draw a clear line."

—Barbara, court-ordered divorce mediator

Your partnership—whether with an estranged ex or a loving spouse—is the model your children will follow. That's why you have to put distance between what angers you and how you respond. Add choice into the equation. If you think this is déjà vu, you're right. We talked about doing this when your children trigger you.

If you choose to take the high road in your partnership, you will help foster emotional security for your children. It's extremely difficult to do in the wake of a painful divorce, but that's probably when it is most important.

"I always felt like my parenting efforts were being undermined by my ex-husband. . . . I try so hard to feed my kids healthy food and not have a lot of screen time. At my ex's house it is like a weekend full of junk food and junk TV.

"After many tearful nights, I decided that since my kids were safe, I was going to adopt the attitude of what happens in Vegas (aka Dad's house) stays in Vegas. When they come home, I have made a ritual of lighting a candle in our entry and hugging them. It helps smooth the transition and lessen the reentry shock."

—Growing mom

"At some point it dawned on me that blaming my ex for all of my unhappiness was getting me nowhere, nor was it helping my kids."

—Divorced mom of three

Even when you know to hold your tongue, it's hard to do. One mom kept a list of questions in mind. "First I would ask myself, 'How will my anger foster my child's growth?' And if that did not work I would ask, 'What would love do? It would

Dump the Trash Talk

- Do not trash talk your partner or ex when your kids are at home. Even if you think they can't hear you, don't risk it. They hear everything.
- Do not trash talk with your body language. Ixnay on the eye rolls and exasperated sighs.
- Stick with the facts, keep your judgments to yourself. Know the difference between reflecting your child's experience and dumping your own.
- Do not make your kids mini detectives. Don't grill them about what happened at Dad's. Even if you are dying to know, don't ask, "What does Daddy's new girlfriend look like?" You're simply inviting disaster.
- Do not compete for your children's affection. No one wins. The goal is to have your child love you both.
- Don't provide running commentary on the other parent's choices. Their house, their rules.
- Progress has never been made through blame.
- Adopt the attitude: I could not change him/her when we lived under the same roof, I certainly don't have the power to do it now.
- Trash talking your ex is trash talking your kid by proxy. It will erode self-esteem.
- Keep asking yourself: How would love talk? What would love do?

make me step back from my anger and try to choose a different response.' "

Whether you're going through a divorce or have a happy marriage, we all have room to download love more purely. Be more tolerant, show respect, have gratitude, choose your words with greater care.

If all else fails and you are ready to let it rip in front of your child, take this mother's long-view advice: "I think twenty years ahead and think about how I would feel if my future daughter-in-law spoke to my son the way that I am speaking to my husband. I would kill her. I guess if my son grows up hearing me nag at my husband 24/7, I have nobody to blame for my future high-maintenance daughter-in-law but myself."

DON'T TRASH TALK YOUR KIDS

Last summer I sat at a long picnic table near a breathtaking mountain. While the parents were eating dinner, the kids ran up a trail in search of a secret fort. Twenty minutes later an exuberant and joyful bunch of seven- and eight-year-olds came running toward the picnic table to share their adventures.

One excited little boy, James, interrupted the adult conversation.

"Mom, Mom, you can't believe what we found!"

Lovingly, his mother smiled and whispered, "I can't wait to hear, James, but grown-ups are talking, and there will be a pause in the conversation. Please wait for the pause."

On my other side, another boy came running up to his mother with equal enthusiasm.

"Mom, Mom, we had so much fun—"

"I am talking! Don't interrupt," she said.

"But, Mom—"

"Be quiet! Can't you see that I am *talking*?"

"But, Mom, we found the—"

"Shut UP, Steve!" she yelled.

My heart sank. I knew what was coming. James, on my right, patiently waited for the pause, enthusiasm still alive and well. Steve, on my left, walked away from the table, looking shamed and dejected, carrying with him stories of secret forts never to be shared.

What opposite responses to the same situation. What markedly different messages to the child! "Wait for the pause" versus "Shut up" gets incorporated so differently into a child's developing sense of self.

"I think of my kids' brains like a computer. I don't want to input data that I won't be able to easily delete later."

—Mother of three

Harsh words reverberate. That's why I want you to promise to eliminate the phrases *Shame on you* or *You should be ashamed* from your vocabulary. Shame becomes internalized self-hatred. I have seen countless patients whose parents' thoughtless words echoed in their heads and chipped away at their self-worth, even decades later.

So we have to discipline ourselves to make our instructions constructive. One great tool is to look for positive behavior to reinforce. Well-behaved children just don't command our attention in the same way whining or disobedient children do. But they should.

Amazing teachers and parents offer the same advice: don't ignore the things that your kids are doing right. Highlight them. Thank your children. Tell them that you noticed how they waited patiently or cleared their plate without being asked. Find things to celebrate and reinforce. The more specific positive reinforcement you use, the more motivated your kids will be. Kids want to please their parents. So catch them doing something right and then give them a big smile and a verbal high five. Chances are they will do it again. Let them feel noticed, appreciated, and valued. There's no better way to shape behavior.

"I always try to choose my words with care. I want to be remembered as a loving leader, not a critical boss."

—Single mom

If you are a critical parent, your kids will take your judgment to heart. Why? Because for the first six years of life, children have trouble sorting reality from imagination, truth from fiction. They rely on you to help them. Children's brain waves are literally in a dreamlike state. This is a fascinating neuroscience fact. They don't know the tooth fairy isn't real or monsters don't exist until you tell them. So if you are calling them naughty, selfish, or lazy, they're probably going to believe you. These words are getting hardwired in when children can't question whether they are true or false. And as children age, what you say about them still matters because they love and respect you.

Careful the things you say, children will listen . . .
Careful the tale you tell, that is the spell . . .
What do you leave to your child when you're dead?
Only whatever you put in its head . . .

—Stephen Sondheim, "Children Will Listen" from *Into the Woods*

Children are listening to your words and also reading your body language. So when you are annoyed, they know. When you pile on the criticism and contempt, the message their developing self gets is: "Look how upset I make my parents, I really bother them." Your eye rolls and negative input will replay over and over.

Don't beat yourself up; we all do this! No parent in the world is constantly patient and always chooses words with grace. But if we practice, good language becomes a habit, and our children internalize a loving voice.

The power of choosing your words mindfully can't be overstated. Words can inspire or deflate, soothe or inflame. "Wait for the pause" increases the likelihood of the child being patient in the future. "Shut up" just leads to shut down.

MODEL HONESTY

Years ago I sat next to an excited girl on a plane. "How old are you?" I asked. "I am five, but for this flight my mom says that I am four. When I get off the plane, my mom says I will be five again."

Trading the truth for a cheaper seat costs so much more in reliability.

Seven-year-old Tony was invited to a Bulls game with his

buddy Jesse. The parking lot was crowded. Jesse's father told the attendant that they had to leave at halftime, so they needed a great parking spot in order to get out. Tony got tearful. When Jesse's dad asked what was wrong, Tony replied, "I have only seen basketball games on TV and I am so sad that we have to leave early." The boy's father said, "Oh, we're staying for the whole game, I was just saying that to get a good parking spot."

It seems harmless enough. But it is shortsighted. Is it really worth the money or minutes you'll save? Think of the message you are telegraphing.

These kinds of strategies come at a big emotional cost. It is tough to shape honesty by modeling deception. Be a trustworthy leader. Actions that match words create safety and strengthen connections.

If you want truthful kids, you have to ditch the white lies and do as don Miguel Ruiz states in his book *The Four Agreements*: "Be impeccable with your word. Speak with integrity. Say only what you mean."

Don Miguel goes on to quote the definition of integrity as a state of wholeness or being unbroken. Think about that. Every time you tell even a tiny lie, you are chipping away at your own wholeness and eroding your self-esteem. It's so much healthier to stay true to yourself in word and deed.

Speak with integrity. And teach your kids to do the same.

DON'T LET YOUR KIDS TRASH TALK

At a restaurant, a young girl spilled her water. Rather than apologizing or wiping up the spill, she turned to her mother and sassed, "You made me!" As I was trying to imagine how that could be, the girl continued. "You made me laugh and that's why I spilled!"

I thought she must be kidding. But her mom knew otherwise and asked her to wipe it up. To which her daughter answered, "You are a mean mommy."

It is very hard to stomach a lack of ownership. Parents are such sticklers for "Please" and "Thank you." And yet "You made me," "I hate you," or "You are a mean mommy" seem to ruffle few parental feathers. In fact, parents often look blasé when children dish out disrespectful commentary.

Do not get me wrong, I am all for self-expression. And for please and thank you. But I am just as adamant about teaching kids ownership. "You made me" is the ultimate abdication of responsibility. Roll it forward. Think of your spouse, friends, or bosses who mess up and say "It is not my fault." Perpetually defensive people who deflect blame turn themselves into victims—powerless to change things for the better. Think of all the grown-up babies whom you know. Do you want your child to become one?

We all make mistakes. Owning them and taking responsibility for them is empowering. Accountability also is quite attractive.

At a Super Bowl party, a nine-year-old went up to his mother and said, "I had a second piece of cake without asking. I am sorry and it won't happen again." A divorced mom overheard and joked, "Does he want to get married?" The boy's mom smiled and answered, "I taught my kids that there is zero shame in making mistakes, just take responsibility for them."

Teach your kids responsibility for their words and actions.

Back in the day, "I hate you" and "You are a mean mommy" would've prompted your parents to wash your mouth out with soap, which makes no sense. Today's parents, wanting to encourage self-expression, value any gem their kid spews. Or, wanting to avoid conflict, they let it slide. Either way, it is sending the message that "whatever comes out of your mouth is OK by me."

I so disagree with the culture that says kids should be able to express their feelings in *any* way. This is part of this crazy pendulum swing. Children used to be fearful of sharing their real emotions with their parents (never a good thing), and now the backlash is that kids can say whatever they want even if they express themselves in inappropriate ways.

Here's the new middle: All feelings are welcome. All expressions of them are not.

Let your kids share all their feelings—without calling names or placing blame. Kids need to let out their anger. In fact, Freud's view was that if you swallow anger long enough, you get depressed. Anger is a defense against hurt. As a parent, you want to get under the heat and down to the hurt. Find out what is really upsetting your children so you can give them the understanding they need. Getting to the root of the problem opens up a channel to a clearer and gentler expression of it.

As soon as you hear "You are a mean mommy," try to name your child's feeling and mirror it back more constructively. "I understand that you are disappointed to have to leave the party, but calling me names is not OK." When you hear "I hate my brother," you can say, "I can tell you're really upset that he took your toy." Address the authentic primary feeling of hurt, not the secondary anger. Redirect the language into more compassionate communication.

Teach your children how to own their mistakes. Banish the *you made me*s. Help them express their feelings in a way that lets them truly be heard—and doesn't put the other person on the defensive. What a priceless gift!

But words are only half of the equation. Tone affects the way your words get heard.

Everyone marvels over Renee's children. A whine never seems to have escaped their lips. When I asked Renee how she pulled that off, she said: "In my house we have a motto: 'Whining gets you nothing.'"

She turned to her kids and asked, "What happens when you whine?" In chorus, they replied, "Whining gets you nothing."

The best part about Renee's policy is her consistent enforcement. She has no tolerance for whining and uses phrases like "I can't hear you when you speak that way." If she cracked down intermittently, it would not be so effective. The consistent reinforcement has completely extinguished whining in her home. How peaceful.

"Speaking with respect is nonnegotiable in my house. I give respect and insist that my kids return the favor."

—Mother of two

LABELS ARE LIMITATIONS

At an outpatient clinic, a psychiatry resident took a new mom's history. During the interview, the mom held her newborn daughter in her arms. "My son is an angel," she said, beaming. "He has been like that since he was born. He is sweet and kind, just a great kid. But my daughter is such a diva. She has trouble written on her forehead. She is going to be a terror in high school."

I had to jump in to clear up my confusion.

"You have three children?" I asked.

"No, just my son and my daughter," she replied.

"Oh, then the diva you are referring to is the baby in your arms?"

Her daughter was only three weeks old and already this mom was writing her unflattering story in permanent Sharpie. The mom was projecting such strong negative feelings onto this peaceful little person. The only way to flip the script was to increase the mother's self-awareness. The resident and I were determined to try.

After some work in therapy, the mom realized that she had a terrible relationship with her own mother and was unconsciously repeating it. She also had trouble with female relationships in general. In therapy she would say women are "complicated, manipulative, and always will disappoint you."

She had to work through her grief over not having the mother she wanted. Then she needed to forgive herself for unwittingly repeating her mom's patterns. Only then could she free herself to be a better mom. With an early intervention and increased self-understanding, the mom blossomed. So, too, did her nondiva daughter.

In an attempt to understand our children—and even to make them feel special—we label them. Some of the labels aren't as harsh as *diva*, but they still stick. My one child is a math whiz, the other is a great reader. One child is so affectionate, the other kid has never been cuddly. Why does it have to be one or the other? Can't someone be good at math AND at reading? Or can't both kids be good at both?

Be curious about any biases that you might have toward your children. Try to see where they come from and how you might let go of them. Labels and comparisons really are no-win. If it is a positive label, kids will always fear losing it. If it is a negative label, someone gets stuck with it.

We have to watch the script that we are writing for our child. My son the angel, my daughter the diva. *And so it is.* What you think about your children skews what you actually see. If you think that your child is lazy, wimpy, impossible, you will look for examples that prove you right. And you will be right. Labels become a self-fulfilling prophecy.

"The way you see people is the way you treat them, and the way you treat them is what they become."

—Johann Wolfgang von Goethe

Labels also put a cap on all that your child can be. But if you drop the labels, you can unleash your child's infinite potential.

"My son got a scholarship to college for football. He was a daisy picker on the field until fourth grade. Flowers bloom when they are ready, and sometimes their blossoms will surprise you."

—East Coast mom

MINIMIZE THE DIVISIONS

A final caution about labels: besides being stifling, they set kids up for sibling rivalry. Comparison breeds competition.

"My mom used to tell my sister that she was the smart one and the pretty one and that I was the creative one. So pretty and smart were already taken? Bummer for me."

—Tales from the couch

Sibling rivalry will find its way into most families. Let's not encourage it by playing favorites or making comparisons. When you make an example out of one child, you create animosity in the other. Saying "See how well your brother is eating his vegetables" doesn't make his sister want to eat hers; it just makes her want to kick him under the table.

Triangulating also fuels sibling rivalry, so try to keep it to a minimum. If you are upset with one child and you tell the other child, all you do is create a bigger drama and never really solve the problem. That's triangulating. Adding another person's emotions to an already charged situation only ups the tension. Problems are best solved face-to-face, one-on-one.

Think about an operating room. Surgeons have sterile procedures to keep patients safe from infection. Families desperately need boundaries to prevent one relationship from infecting another. So keep a boundary; don't share your woes about one child with his or her siblings. Keep your issues with each of your children separate from their relationships with each other.

On the other hand, when stitching two families together, make sure the words you use do not cut anyone out. The language of blended families is often unintentionally alienating.

"When I remarried and had my second son, my older son kept saying, 'Ryan is my half brother.' I told him that Ryan was the only brother that he was getting and that we did not use the word half *in our family. 'I know that it is hard to imagine, but that guy in diapers is your brother and buddy for life and will most likely be the best man in your wedding.' "*

—Merged-family mom

Over the years I have encouraged my outpatients to trade "This is my daughter and my stepson" for "This is my family." If you have a vision of being one family, use words that make everyone feel included.

Skip the half and be whole.

FIND YOUR FIT

Even though you want to lay off the labels, you still need to recognize that each of your children is different and respond accordingly. One size does not fit all in parenting; tailor your parenting to fit your child.

"I have two very different sons. My older son is critical of himself; he will have played a great football game and then beat himself up for one play. I always point out to him how many things he did right. My younger son has the opposite

problem. He once told me that he had scored all four touchdowns and had won the game for his team. I asked him if he thought that one of his teammates was blocking so that he could score and if one of his buddies threw him the pass that he scored the winning touchdown with."

—Father of three

Anyone who has more than one child will attest to how different siblings can be. The parenting strategies that worked so well for one child can fail miserably on the second.

I am going to out an uncomfortable secret. Some kids are simply a better temperamental fit for a particular parent. A better organic match between parent and child makes bonding easier. The strong attachment forms almost effortlessly. A less harmonious match—or a painfully familiar reflection—can make parenting more challenging.

"I am very shy and my oldest daughter has always been very social and carefree. I get such a kick out of her. My other daughter is cautious and extremely shy. It is very tough for me to watch her interact. When we are at the park I want to yell, 'Play, don't just watch the other kids play.' It's hard for me to parent her. We are yin meets yin. I am better when yin meets yang."

—Self-aware dad

Chemistry between people is that intangible *X* factor. Somehow we think it is going to be natural when it comes to our children. Because they are ours, we should fit seamlessly. Wouldn't that be nice? Accepting reality helps us adjust our parenting styles to meet our kids. Even—or especially—when mismatched temperaments make bonding difficult, it is important to be curious about your own biases so that children don't feel your judgments of them. Our judgments get in the way of really connecting.

At the bus stop every morning, I observed an uncomfortable, but very common, dynamic: a mom who clearly lit up when addressing one of her daughters, but not the other.

"Jamie, sweet pea, have a great day! See you, Tara." That send-off communicates everything a child needs to know. And it just got worse when they got back off the bus. Mom smiled and rushed up to kiss Jamie, then said "hey" and gave a pat to Tara.

Watching this splitting dynamic was becoming more painful every day. I do not normally practice bus stop therapy, but this mom gave me an opening, and I took it. Turns out, I didn't have to say much.

"Jamie is so cuddly, sweet, and easy, but Tara has always been tough," the mom said after the bus pulled away. "She's so negative. To be totally honest, she bugs me."

"I see the way you light up when you look at Jamie," I observed.

"Yes." Her mother gleamed.

"I bet Jamie sees that glimmer when you look at her with so much love," I said.

Fortunately, this woman was a very quick study. "So you think Tara knows that she does not make me light up in the same way?"

The mom, filled with remorse, answered her own question: "Yes, of course she does! How do I change this?" Again, she answered herself: "I know, I am going to fake it until I make it. I am not going to say one critical thing about Tara for a week. I am going to take her out for a dinner alone. I have never done that with her."

What a turnaround! It was so heartwarming to watch the dynamic change over the next several months. At first Tara looked confused by the change, unsure that she could trust it. But after a few months, Tara would get on the bus, smiling back at her mom, knowing the love was being reflected right back at her. How great to know we can change our ways and undo earlier damage.

Kids live to see the twinkle in their parents' eye. It makes them feel cherished and adored. Make sure you discover that special quality in each child that makes you light up.

Study your child with your heart, not just your head.

NO TRASH TALKING YOURSELF OR YOUR BODY

A mother was playing with her five- and seven-year-old daughters. The girls were laughing and joking with her. It was a sweet scene. One of the girls lifted up her mom's shirt to tickle her tummy. The mother's flat belly looked like an airbrushed magazine ad. Yet she quickly pulled down her shirt.

"Don't show everyone my fat stomach," she snapped.

I was shocked on two levels: first at her own distorted body image, and worse yet at the loud message that she was telegraphing to her little girls.

If we talk about our bodies in a critical way, we teach our kids to do the same. Talking about your own flaws unintentionally holds a magnifying glass to theirs. You may not connect the dots, but, I promise you, your kids do.

"I remember that as a teenager I asked my mom why she never wore sleeveless shirts, and she said, 'Oh, I could never go sleeveless, my arms are too fat.' I remember looking in the mirror that night thinking, Do I have fat arms?"

—Tales from the couch

One mom had three children with more olive complexions and one lighter-skinned son. She would innocently say to the fair-skinned child, "Dad and I have dark skin. I wonder how you got such fair skin?" One day the mom was applying sunscreen to her lighter-skinned child and he asked her to stop. He wanted his skin to get darker. Unintentionally, she had been telling him, "You are not like us"—which he took to mean "less than." The mom immediately realized her mistake. "Sweetheart," she said, "I want you to wear sunscreen so that you can protect your beautiful fair skin that I love so much."

We can help our children to feel more comfortable in their own skin if we think of our words as sunscreen protecting their developing psyches.

YOUR THOUGHTS ARE THE FINAL FRONTIER

Try to be as compassionate with yourself as you would be with your children. Positive self-talk—and limiting negative self-talk—are critical to mental health.

A patient once said, "I knew that I had to change, because I would never let someone else talk to me the way I was talking to myself."

If you continually talk to yourself with fear statements, you may get anxious; if you talk to yourself with self-critical statements, you can become depressed. I'm oversimplifying, but neuroscience backs this up. We know that positive thoughts carry positive neurochemistry, while negative thoughts are depleting. Good thoughts can actually raise your serotonin, which makes you calmer and happier.

"One of the most significant findings in psychology research in the last twenty years is that individuals can choose the way they think."

—Martin Seligman, PhD, founder of positive psychology

Teach your kids to program a kinder, gentler narration into their heads, and how to change the channel when the conversation turns negative. You would jump on your children if they called their friends stupid; be as vigilant when they call themselves stupid or other derogatory terms.

In one great teacher's class, the rule is "You can't say, 'I don't get this.' You can say, 'I don't get this YET.' 'I don't get this YET' is the difference between giving up and believing in yourself. I insist on this small change, as it represents a big change in the psychology of how you see yourself. It helps to write a different story."

"Our life is shaped by our mind; we become what we think."

—Buddha

A high school basketball player felt like his performance was letting his team down. He became more stressed-out and frustrated with each move. The more he criticized himself, the worse his game got. After halftime, he did a 180, and his basketball followed his attitude. When his dad asked how he did it, he said, "When I kept telling myself that I was playing badly, it made me more tense and I played worse. I decided to be gentle with the mental. Instead of beating myself up, I cut myself some mental slack. I told myself, 'Move on, next ball, no worries.' "

Limiting negative narration is always a game changer, in sports or in life.

There is a whole psychology field, called cognitive behavioral therapy, devoted to this very thing. Change your thoughts and you can change your feelings and your behavior. Thoughts vibrate with energy, good or bad. Therefore, how we talk to ourselves influences much of our mental health.

So go ahead, push delete on the negative internal chatter. Replace critical thoughts with more loving ones. This requires practice. But the payoff is huge. When you rehearse these skills, your brain function actually improves and you boost your happiness. Teach yourself loving, compassionate self-talk and then pass it on to your kids.

A Cherokee legend tells of a grandfather teaching his grandson by the fire.

" 'Inside me, there is a fight raging between two wolves. One wolf is anger, bitterness, self-pity, jealousy, and sorrow.

The other wolf is love, faith, hope, peace, forgiveness, and joy. Both wolves are strong, and they battle fiercely—not just in me, but in everyone, even you.'

"The young boy thought for a moment and asked, 'Grandfather, which wolf will win?'

"The wise elder replied, 'The one you feed.'"

Shrink Notes

Trash the Trash Talk

1. Trash talking your ex or partner is trash talking your kid by proxy. Skip the verbal and nonverbal trash talk.
2. Choose mindful language. Negative narrations are hard to shake.
3. Replace critical self-talk with compassionate self-talk.
4. Accentuate the positive; point out things that your kids are doing right.
5. Teach your kids how to express their feelings without blame or name-calling.
6. Get under the heat and down to the hurt.
7. Teach your kids to own their mistakes. It is the difference between being a victim and being empowered. Banish "You made me."
8. Label your files, not your kids. Labels are limitations.
9. Watch the data that you are inputting into your child's head. It will outlast you.
10. Ask yourself: Can I say this same thing with more love?

CHAPTER SIX

Prada Kids

Is there really a human race? Is it going on now all over the
place?
Do I warm up and stretch? Do I practice and train?
Do I get my own coach? Do I get my own lane? . . .
Shouldn't it be that you just try your best?
And that's more important than beating the rest?
Shouldn't it be looking back at the end
That you judge your own race by the help that you lend?

—Jamie Lee Curtis, *Is There Really a Human Race?*

I received a call from a man whose daughter was accepted a year early to a "highly sought-after kindergarten." Because she would be younger than most of her classmates, he called me for advice on whether to hold her back a year or to let her start in the fall. He sounded anxious, so I asked him what he was concerned about. He said, "Bottom line: Will this decision be the difference between a stripper pole or admission to Yale?"

We both laughed, knowing that behind the joke was real concern. Parents today agonize over every decision. Every move has to be masterfully orchestrated to prevent any early misstep from knocking your child out of the Fortune 500 or the NBA. Boy, do we feel powerful.

Anxiety today is palpable and pervasive. We are consumed with the delusion that we can line up our children's future. Sadly, our myopic focus on achievement blocks our ability to see our children in all their glory. We are so fixated on our goals for them that we are blinded to their real needs.

So much parental emphasis on "winning" can make love feel conditional. Believing you will only love them "if" breeds insecurity instead of making them feel wholly loved.

As professional women have become professional moms, they, along with dads, have brought professional expectations about performance to parenting. These skill sets just don't translate. The very skills that help you succeed in the workplace collide with the essences of childhood. Work is scheduled, competitive, orderly, fast-paced. Childhood is slow, messy, unfolding without deadlines and spreadsheets.

Trying to impose a worklike order drains the fun out of parenting. Parenting becomes a project, not a relationship. And then childhood is about performance, not just being a well-loved, carefree kid.

By defining success as good grades and trophies received, we are getting in the way of real child development. We are beefing up children's external résumés at the expense of their internal selves. We are creating fragile egos instead of building self-esteem. We have it all backward.

"We are all guilty of expecting way too much of our children. We say we just want our kids to be happy, but we mean we want them to be happy living our definition of success."

—Elementary school administrator

Childhood was not meant to withstand this pressure. I worry about the little psyches subjected to the sheer force of this premature stress.

Parents who hover, micromanage, and overschedule look so involved. But when we are laser-focused on performance, we risk the most essential part of childhood development: making a real connection.

"It used to be that children were seen and not heard, and now today's kids are heard and hovered over—and yet we are still not really seeing children. Today's parents want a perfect child. You can have Prada boots, but today's parents want Prada kids."

—Lisette Davison, MD, child psychiatrist

In spending so much time trying to make kids perfect and give them a leg up on the competitive world, we are compromising their mental health. Setting high standards for a child is great; obsessing over performance just creates anxiety. Let's give our kids their childhood back. Our unconditional love for them and our deep connection to them is the best leg up. But this generation has confused hovering with love.

"It is not attention that a child is seeking, but love."

—Sigmund Freud

When hovering becomes extreme it turns into interference. Injecting yourself into your children's every activity prevents them from gaining competence. If you take it on yourself to correct the papers and stack the team with ringers, your children are never going to learn how to get anything done on their own or discover their own passions. Self-reliance seems out of fashion, but it should never be passé. It is critical to child development. As are coping skills. But we've taken them out of the equation, too, and then thrown kids headfirst into high-pressure academics and sports. We have created a perfect storm for combustion.

And we are laying on this pressure in the hopes of controlling what cannot be controlled. We are under the mistaken notion that we can engineer our children's future. It's like being the white-knuckled passenger on an airplane. All the gripping of your seat and pushing imaginary brakes with your feet will not make the plane land safely. Your children's future, in many ways, is the same. Jockey all you want, they may not get into the college of their choice. Or yours. So many valedictorians get rejected every year. So few outstanding students get academic scholarships. Even fewer high school athletes go on to play in college, much less the pros.

Put your efforts where they matter most—developing a deep and loving relationship with your child and fostering great character.

PRADA ACADEMICS

We are parenting on Red Bull. Our anxiety is so endemic that we've managed to roll college pressure back to embryonic development.

"I feel as if I am a bad mom. I never played music to my child when I was pregnant. I just read on the Internet that you could stimulate your child and even increase IQ points if they were listening to soothing music while you're pregnant. I feel guilty I didn't do this for my kid."

—Mother of a one-year-old

Moms worry too much even before their kids are born. What many of them don't know is that anxiety is the bigger risk factor for a developing fetus or growing child. At the Women's Life Center at UCLA, we treat depression and anxiety during pregnancy to keep these mood disorders from compromising fetal health. For this particular woman, lessening her anxiety would pay far greater dividends than playing Mozart—in utero and out.

But anxiety is in the ethos, and parents worry that they are not measuring up. It starts with music during pregnancy, then flash cards and educational videos in infancy. The notion that watching videos can increase intelligence flies in the face of science. In fact, pediatricians recommend no screen time for children under the age of two. (For me, that's still too young.) Neurons in the brain are stimulated when parents and infants interact. Responding to the cues of your newborn—mirroring them, cooing, stroking—lights up your baby's brain in a way a passive screen never could.

We have misunderstood how learning really takes place in these early years. Interactive human experience, which engages all the senses, will always trump a consumer product. We have sold ourselves a bill of goods, believing that our priority as parents is to give children an academic edge. We've been sidetracked from the real heart of parenthood: creating a safe and loving connection with our children. This is the best head start program that any parent can offer!

But big business fuels misconceptions and preys on parental worries. A commercial for a learning center depicts information spilling out of a child's brain over summer vacation. Message: forget riding a bike or swimming in a lake; kids need to be drilling facts over the summer or they will lose everything they ever learned. Funny, I don't remember learning about a flip-top in the brain when I was in medical school.

We are parenting out of fear, not faith. Marketers take advantage of those concerns, making moderate parenting a challenge. Look at the not-so-subtle names of some actual learning centers:

One Step Ahead [Who wants to be a step behind?]
First to Learn [We could be second? Oh, no!]
Right Start [Did I give my kid the wrong start?]

I hear so many parents of toddlers tell me, "I fear that if I don't do all of this stuff, my kids will get behind." Behind what? Get a grip. Your kid still sleeps in a Onesie.

Every teacher that I interviewed said parents have wildly unrealistic expectations of perfect academic records from the get-go.

"Kids are not perfect little people, they should not be college-ready in second grade."

—Elementary school teacher

"Kindergarten is the new first grade and high school is the new college. . . . It is just nuts! Parents want their kids to get a perfect report card and are panic-stricken when they don't get it. Did the parents themselves get straight A's? Did any teacher teaching them have straight A's? We are expecting way too much from children. . . . Our school had to call in a psychologist to instruct the teachers how to deal with all of the anxiety that we are seeing."

—Elementary school educator

Too much pressure and stress is not good for any adult, much less a growing child. Medically speaking, stress triggers a fight-or-flight response. Sensing danger, your sympathetic nervous system starts to secrete adrenaline and cortisol. The heart races, your blood pressure rises, and your muscles tighten, all preparing you to run for your life. Helpful if you are trying to outrun a bear. Less so if you are studying for a test.

Stress affects our bodies and brains whether the stressor is physical or psychological. A little stress can boost performance, but chronic, daily stress wreaks havoc. It can actually shrink a part of your brain (the hippocampus) where memory resides. It can increase headaches, cause ulcers, decrease immune function and trigger autoimmune disease, and so forth. Stress also worsens all psychiatric illnesses.

Obviously this is not our goal when we're trying to get our kids to do well in school. But we have to be careful and not turn our children into performance monkeys.

"Sometimes I think that my parents have mistaken me for a superhero or a robot. I feel constant pressure to be perfect at everything."

—High school student

"I feel that I have spent my high school career performing and preparing myself to look good for colleges, signing up for activities not because I like them, but because maybe some future admissions officer will."

—High school senior

Parents are just too enmeshed in their children's academics. A mom asked another mother to go out to dinner. The friend answered, "I wish I could, we are just so buried in college applications." The first mom thought, Who is *we*? Another mother called a law professor to complain about her son's grade. In *law school*! Is she going to dispute the bar exam for him, too?

We are teaching our children that they need us in order to succeed, that they cannot do the work without us. This creates dependency. When parents overfunction, kids underfunction.

When Mommy talks to your teacher about your grade or Daddy refutes your essay question, you do not build the skills to do it for yourself. Children need to handle things on their own. When parents do everything for children, they create psychological fragility. Let's not swoop in early to try to fix everything.

"In the last ten years I've had to give a speech to the parents of the new freshman class, begging parents to get out of their children's way. 'I am going to turn your boys into men, but

only if you let me. Don't e-mail the teachers. Don't correct the papers. Let's make a pact together not to shield our kids from the very experiences that build strength of character.'"

—Catholic school teacher

Instead of building our children's strength, we treat them like babies—as shrinks say, infantilize them—and then expect them to function like mini-adults. We are piling on pressure without ever having given them the psychological resilience to manage it. How can they handle three advance placement classes if we don't allow them to tolerate a little cookie dough in their ice cream?

Here's a cautionary tale. I recently saw a "Prada kid" for evaluation. Stacy's parents had given her every "advantage"—every tutor, every enrichment class, and tons of "attention" since preschool.

"I think I started feeling really anxious in fifth grade," she told me, "but my parents were so proud of my report cards and my swimming success that I did not want to disappoint them by telling them how I felt inside."

Stacy, her parents, and her team of tutors had gained her admission to one of the most prestigious Ivy League schools in the country. I saw her after debilitating anxiety and depression forced her to drop out.

All of this pressure is backfiring. Depression, anxiety, substance abuse, and suicide rates among children and teens are on the rise. More parents are turning to psychiatrists for help. If they came to me, I would suggest starting with environmental changes such as reducing academic load, increasing free time, and prioritizing family time. This could go a long way toward helping our children find the balance they so desperately need.

Unfortunately, rather than rethinking their priorities and getting to the source of the stress, many parents and students simply request medication—even when it is not indicated. When needed for attention-deficit/hyperactivity disorder, stimulant medications can make an enormous difference in a patient's quality of life. But these days, ADHD medications are being requested as "study drugs." Here is where we have to draw the line.

On any given night in an East Coast college library, stimulants can be had for eight dollars a pill, several students told me. One student explained their potency:

"Kids are literally selling them in the library. I am a senior and have never tried drugs and I don't take any medications. But it was finals and I was really tired, so I bought one. It was amazing! I became one with my book. I stayed up until three A.M. and I was wide-awake and insanely focused. I jammed on my chemistry test and thought, Wow, if I had taken this all the way through, I could have been summa cum laude."

I asked her how stimulants like Adderall are so readily available. She said that students Google the symptoms of ADHD, then report them to psychiatrists so they will prescribe the drugs. She said that kids are very casual about using and selling medications.

"Over a four-year collegiate experience, almost two-thirds of students are offered prescription stimulants for nonmedical use."

—"Nonmedical Use of Prescription Stimulants During College," *Journal of American College Health*, March 2012

Abuse of prescription medication is no small thing. Stimulants can cause anxiety, mood swings, heart palpitations, decrease in appetite, and trouble sleeping. Doctors take careful medical histories and sometimes recommend tests to rule out cardiac illness before prescribing stimulants. I am sure there are no EKG machines at the library.

Stimulants increase dopamine in your brain, and excessive dopamine can cause psychosis. Psychosis is a break with reality. We have broken with reality as a culture if we are using these drugs when they are not medically indicated! Stimulants can reduce appetite and sleep, two essential components for a healthy growing body. You can lose up to an inch of height. Using them to get into, or succeed in, college is shortsighted and irresponsible.

But students don't think like that. I asked a Hamilton College senior if kids worried about the harmful effects of stimulant use.

"When was the last time you met a college student who made a decision based on what's good for their body?" she said, laughing.

That's why they need parents to remember the big picture and not get roped into fostering drug dependence.

"We routinely test college athletes for steroid use; are we now going to have to do drug tests on students in the libraries and dorm rooms to deal with unfair academic edge?"

—Concerned dad

Ironically, all this "academic edge" is undermining the very self-esteem we want to build. Consider the warped psychology in kids thinking they need medication to perform. We need to teach them to rely on themselves, not on substances.

A recent college grad jokingly asked me for stimulant medication. "I am so used to taking it for school, how am I going to focus for twelve-hour workdays without it?"

This has to stop.

We need to back off building our kids' résumés and go back to simply being with and enjoying our children. Show your kids how deeply loved and accepted they are without pressuring them to perform.

Instead of being so invested in the outcome of our kids' learning, we need to let them enjoy the process of learning for its own sake. Encourage discovery by letting them play, explore, and have the time to dream.

I heard Yong Zhao, a Chinese educator, say at a conference that China outperforms America on test scores by a large margin. But when it comes to innovation and leadership, he added, "We are still waiting for our Steve Jobs."

In other words, excessive homework, overscheduling, and rote memorization may create worker bees, but it is less likely to build a future entrepreneur. Nor is it the formula for your child's psychological well-being.

Let's remind ourselves that a perfect transcript and hundreds of hours of "enrichment" activities do not guarantee anything. They certainly don't keep your child out of a shrink's office. Therapists across the country see countless patients who look great on paper but feel empty on the inside.

If trophies and good grades were the formula for self-esteem, many therapists would be out of business. We need to catch our collective breath and lose the "my kid is getting behind" mentality. Let's make home a respite from, not a continuation of, the pressures of school and sports.

One mom realized that her two children were taking themselves way too seriously. Both were hypercritical of their mistakes and starting to develop perfectionist tendencies. Out of concern, she founded the Slovenly Club. Every night at dinner she and her husband would share their biggest mess-ups of the day. Soon her kids followed suit. They would compare their mistakes and rate each other, and the largest flub of the day would be heralded as the winner. Laughter erupted as the kids competed with gusto for the Slovenly Award. The now-grown kids found the club so entertaining—and so freeing—that they preside over Slovenly Clubs at their own dinner tables.

Embracing mistakes liberates children to take risks and try new things. If they make mistakes, they know they can bounce back—and reach new heights. If you still feel compelled to keep driving and pushing your kids, take a lesson from these parents. They know it's OK to ease off.

"In today's perform, perform schools, I try to help my daughter get perspective by telling her that it is better to be good at life than good at school."

—West Coast mother

"I grew up watching endless hours of Lost in Space *and now I am a brain surgeon."*

—Chicago dad

"I am aiming for my kids to be really mediocre, not just a little mediocre. When all of these superkids burn out, my kids will just be getting started."

—Connecticut mother of three

PRADA SPORTS

Hit the stands of any athletic field today and you really see how hard kids are pushed. Sports used to be about fresh air, exercise, teamwork, and just plain fun. They burned off energy and stress. Now they are every bit the pressure cooker school is, as parents try to engineer college scholarships on preschool playing fields.

Again, our intentions start out honorably. We think we are showing our love by being involved in ways our parents never were. Looks good at first glance. But if parents could really see and hear themselves, and understand the toll the win-at-all-costs mentality is taking on their kids, they might call a time-out.

First, the physical price: many orthopedic surgeons are seeing an increase in injuries from organized sports for young kids. Meanwhile, recreational sports injuries are dropping.

"Maybe one message is: just let them go out and play," Dr. Shital Parikh told the *Cincinnati Enquirer*. "You don't have to get them in organized sports at a very young age."

Another physician echoed this concern.

"We are seeing many overuse injuries in kids. I treat kids with Little League elbow. Parents would never let their kid

in a car without a car seat and yet they allow them to pitch endless balls with an injured elbow or shoulder."

—Andrew Weiss, MD, orthopedic surgeon

And that's just the physical injuries. Think of the wear and tear on kids' psyches.

At a basketball game, I once saw the loveliest Dad Jekyll turn into Coach Hyde when his eight-year-old players were down twelve baskets in the fourth quarter.

"Do you kids want to be WINNERS or LOSERS?" he screamed. "Right now you look like losers!"

The devastated look on his son's face showed the pain his father was unwittingly inflicting. Language like that bruises. Instead of inspiring and building up these eight-year-olds' confidence, the coach was basically telling them that if they don't win THIS game, they are losers in life. And they were eight!

After another game, I saw a dad walking fifteen feet in front of his son, berating him for what he could have done differently. The kid absorbed a more damaging message: "Dad will withdraw love if I don't play well." How much better it would have been if this dad walked by his son's side and asked how he felt about the game. Stop grooming children for a sporting career that's highly unlikely. Invest in the person they can become, not the star athlete you envision.

Our messages to kids—even other people's kids—are so loaded. At a basketball game, I sat next to a mom who cheered loudly when the opposing team got called for traveling or committing a foul. Then it got even uglier. The gym grew quiet as a nervous little ten-year-old approached the free-throw line.

Breaking the silence, this woman started screaming: "MISS! MISS!"

What kind of sportsmanship are we modeling here? Look, everybody loves to win. It's fun! Competition can fuel a desire to try hard and to improve. But we have confused competition with a mandate to WIN. And it's had a horrible effect on the behavior of children and of parents. I have witnessed dads shoving each other over their kids' soccer games. I have seen parents get kicked out of games for berating refs. I've seen too many kids' joy turn to sadness over their parents' bad behavior.

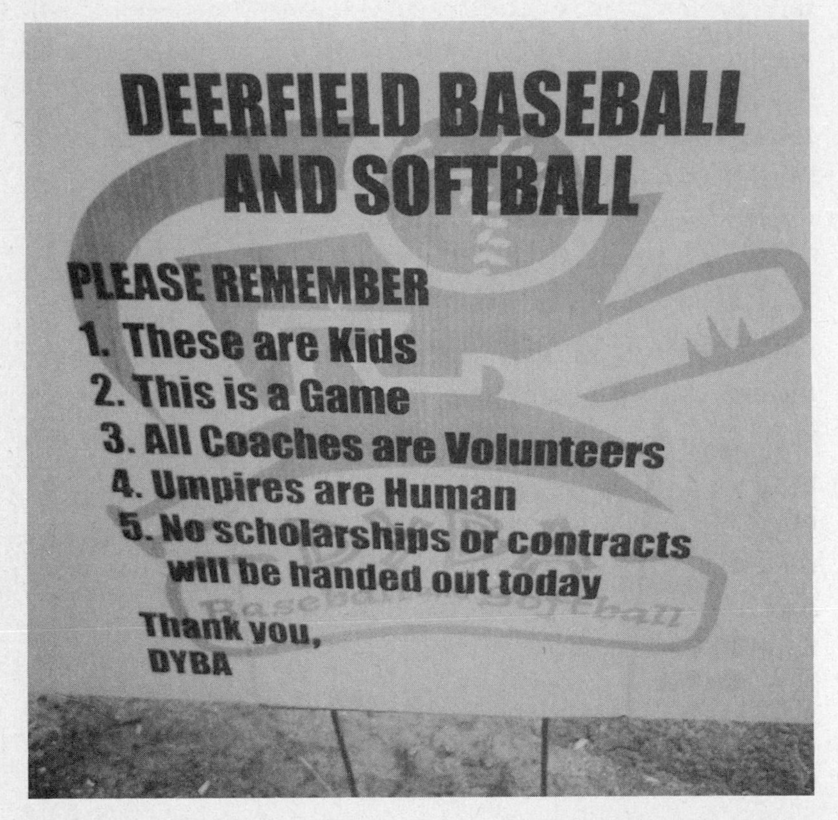

ACTUAL PHOTO FROM A YOUTH BALLPARK IN DEERFIELD, ILLINOIS

Let's get some perspective. Looking back from a shrink's couch one day, what do you think these children will remember: the score of any given game or seeing their dad get into a fight? Children need parents to balance their passions, not inflame them.

"We're modeling crazy from the sidelines."

—Father of two

We're not behaving any better behind the scenes. A California dad went to the draft for his eight-year-old's flag football team. He was shocked to see the fierce arguments over players, and fathers sitting their kids out or having them tank the tryouts so other coaches wouldn't know how good they were. "I could not believe what I was seeing," he told me. "Parents were rigging the draft for eight-year-olds!"

There is a huge difference between being involved in kids' lives and being so invested in kids' winning that parents are willing to cheat. We're undermining the very moral development we are supposed to be building! And stacking the deck isn't a real win anyway. Winning by cheating doesn't foster self-esteem any more than handing out trophies for just showing up does. When kids work hard and genuinely earn a victory, they feel a sense of accomplishment that they can fall back on when future tasks get difficult. When trophies are handed out as parting gifts, or when parents cheat their way to a win, kids are cheated out of the satisfaction of triumph. As I said before, self-esteem comes in part from mastery, from feeling your own competence. That's the real prize.

But our egos get in the way. Kids are not shiny objects

that reflect us; they have their own soul story. We cannot help them develop that story when we're so consumed with projecting our own onto them.

"Parents are so busy living vicariously through their kids, it blocks their good judgment."

—Father of three

"We want a do-over for our own childhood. Is this really about our kids or is it more about us?"

—Cara Natterson, MD, pediatrician and author

It goes back to our Prada kids. We're trying to engineer perfect grades and victories to line up college scholarships. Never mind how unlikely that is. Never mind all the good stuff our kids—and we parents—are missing out on in the meantime. Never mind that this is not the recipe for mental health.

One dad was visibly distraught after his son's team lost a game.

"I am upset for my son," he told me. "He hates losing!"

I glanced at the ten-year-old. He was having a blast, laughing and joking with his buddy. Let's be clear who cared about losing. We have to stop seeing our kids through the lens of our own agenda.

Remember that love is being seen and known and accepted. If this dad continues to project his feelings onto his child, he will miss out on his son's experience and his son's perspective. That just builds walls where you want to build relationships. Similarly, tying performance to lovability makes love feel conditional. It's a message they pick up early.

One first grader, when asked what made him feel loved, answered: "When my mom kisses and hugs me. And with my dad? When I win at sports."

Imagine feeling like you have to win to get love at age six.

Love that is *unconditional* is what gives children real confidence and self-esteem. They know they are loved for who they are, not for living up to some arbitrary standard. Having to perform to please your parents makes you have to swallow a part of your authentic self. That erodes the parent-child bond and undermines a child's sense of identity.

> *"My senior year, I started to ask myself, 'Do I even like volleyball? Did I ever? Or was this really about making my dad happy? Do I have to keep playing in college out of guilt to make all of his time worthwhile?'"*
>
> —Former high school athlete

Imagine how much less she would have struggled if her parents had dropped their agendas and met her where she was.

> *"Great parents are respectful, involved but not intrusive. When the kids' interest shift, the parents shift with them."*
>
> —Josh Anderson, Kansas Teacher of the Year

One mother's aha moment came after she really tuned into her seven-year-old son.

"I had been driving him all over town to get him to his games. At one game, instead of chatting with the other moms, I just watched him play. It dawned on me that he did not look like he was having fun. So on the way home I asked him if he even liked basketball. He said, 'I really do, Mom. I just don't like it when I get the ball. I like basketball except for the ball part.' I laughed and thought, We won't be signing up next season."

—St. Louis mother of two

Parents think that participating in sports will help kids feel good about themselves and teach them to thrive in competitive settings. But if the kids aren't interested, they aren't going to feel good about what they are doing. If you set aside what you think they should be doing and really study your children with your heart, you can find out who *they* are and what *they* love.

"I, too, fell into the trap of thinking that early sports would turn my kid into a great athlete, so I signed Paul up for soccer when he was four. I was really excited for his first game until I saw him chasing a butterfly instead of kicking the ball. I screamed, 'Get in the game, Paul!' What was I doing? He was one year out of diapers! Shouldn't he be chasing butterflies?"

—Philadelphia mom

It's so amazing when realization dawns. But some parents need help for that lightbulb to turn on. If we pay attention, our children often will illuminate the path.

I watched an overinvolved dad scream at his twelve-year-old son, Jeffrey, calling out play-by-play instructions from the top of the stands: "What are you *doing*? Send the ball! Shoot! No, that is the wrong play!" Then he buried his head in his hands in frustration. His negativity was so distracting, it was hard for me to focus on the game. I wondered how Jeffrey was even able to concentrate. Apparently, he wasn't.

Jeffrey called for a time-out, then walked into the stands and said to his father: "Can you please stop, Dad? You are embarrassing me. This is not the NBA, this is twelve-year-old basketball."

You tell 'em, kid!

Another dad, Craig, regretted never having any formal tennis lessons as a kid and did not want his daughter to miss out. So he decided to take Kelly to the park to teach her tennis. After a month of hitting balls every weekend, six-year-old Kelly asked, "Dad, why do you need me to play tennis?"

She might as well have hit the ball right at his head. Craig quickly realized that tennis was more about his own unmet need, not his daughter's. Then he lobbed a winner. "What would you like to do at the park?" he asked. Kelly's face lit up. "How about tag?"

If we are receptive to growing ourselves, our children can lead us where we need to go. An assist from a great coach always helps.

Tracy, a former college athlete, grew tired of trying to coach girls' soccer against persistent parental interference. When her repeated appeals to quit coaching from the bleachers got no traction, she kicked into high gear. She called a Saturday morning practice and told the parents to come dressed in sweats and sneakers. She told the moms and dads to take the field and the team to take the stands, with extra instructions for the kids to act like their parents at their games. The minute the parents got on the field, the kids began screaming, "Kick the ball! Run! Come on! Get in there! Move your feet! What are you DOING?"

The girls had a blast. It was cathartic for them and eye-opening for their parents. And it was very gratifying for Tracy. "At the next game, as the parents were about to scream, you could see them stop and catch themselves and even laugh. Finally they got it!" They got what their kids had known all along. It was not the parents' game. It never was their game. That time had passed. They needed to back away and let their kids have their own experience and discover their own athleticism.

"Parents need to let the game breathe. Kids today are so overcoached that they have lost their own natural instincts. Kids learn most when no one is there to teach them. Parents are too close to their kids' athletic experience. It is not the kids today who are so different, it is the parents."

—Sue Enquist, Hall of Fame softball coach

Parents today seem to have taken Malcolm Gladwell's Outliers too literally. Gladwell's book says the key to success in any task is practicing for ten thousand hours. Even if that works, it's not a prescription for a balanced childhood. Or a balanced brain. Research shows that when you keep practicing things you are already good at, your brain develops so much more in that area that it becomes lopsided. Doing things at which you don't excel naturally strengthens the less-developed parts of your brain. That's why it is so critical for kids growing up to sample a whole variety of activities and subjects.

Date	Day	Type	Start Time	End Time	Field
Jun-7	Thursday	Practice	6:00 PM	8:15 PM	Field B
Jun-8	Friday	Practice	3:30 PM	5:45 PM	Field A
Jun-9	Saturday	Practice	11:00 AM	1:00 PM	Field A
Jun-10	Sunday	Practice	4:00 PM	6:15 PM	Field B
Jun-11	Monday	Practice	6:00 PM	8:15 PM	Field B
Jun-13	Wednesday	Warm-up	4:45 PM	5:30 PM	Field A Cages
Jun-13	Wednesday	Game	6:00 PM	8:30 PM	Field A
Jun-14	Thursday	Practice	6:00 PM	8:15 PM	Field B
Jun-15	Friday	Game	6:30 PM	8:30 PM	Field A
Jun-16	Saturday	Practice	11:00 AM	1:00 PM	Field A
Jun-17	Sunday	Practice	6:00 PM	8:15 PM	Field A
Jun-18	Monday	Practice	6:00 PM	8:15 PM	Field B
Jun-20	Wednesday	Practice	6:00 PM	8:15 PM	Field B
Jun-21	Thursday	Game	6:30 PM	8:30 PM	Field A
Jun-22	Friday	Practice	6:00 PM	8:15 PM	Field B

ACTUAL EIGHT-YEAR-OLD'S BASEBALL SCHEDULE

An Oregon dad flipped Gladwell's script.

"I love sports. I was a college athlete. But when I looked at the baseball schedule for my nine-year-old, it seemed comical to me. I did not want to take the love of any game away from my son, so we did not sign up for organized sports the following spring.

"I decided to take the time I was going to put into coaching and instead bring my son and his buddies to the park. I brought balls and bats, footballs and soccer balls, and sat on the bench and watched them play. When they

asked for help, which was not often, I would jump in. I struggled with thinking that by today's standard my kid was 'getting behind,' and I knew I was taking away ten thousand hours of practice, but I was giving him back those ten thousand hours to be a child. And I knew in my heart, I was doing the right thing."

—Roger, dad

CHARACTER

"I dream of the day when children are praised for being kind, considerate, caring human beings, and not only for their academic, athletic, or financial achievements. That, to me, is a world truly worth dreaming about."

—Steven Carr Reuben, PhD, *Children of Character*

There's your big picture. Kindness, compassion, and character are the keys to a life well lived. These eternal qualities are much more valuable than any athletic victory or academic A's. The two things parents have the best chance to influence are connection and character. Trophies may come and go, grades may rise and fall, but connection and character are your child's to keep.

So how do we inculcate character? By reinforcing it. When you see moments of character, talk about them. Give enthusiastic praise when your children are kind and do the right thing. Talk up others who do the same. And, above all, model ethical choices yourself. Make sure your kids know that character is not about getting praise for something. It is about doing the right thing even when no one is watching. That's when you really feel good about yourself and really feel whole. That is an enormous part of self-esteem.

A boy and his friend were competing to win first place in their elementary school's mile run. The winner would have his name on the gym's wall. Joe and Jack were neck and neck rounding the last lap. Joe tripped, and Jack realized that he was wide open to cross the finish line. Instead Jack stopped and helped his friend up, knowing it would cost him first place. Another kid flew by to win. But Jack had won a much bigger prize. He had proven himself to be a kind and compassionate friend. Now, that's a win.

So is exercising ethics. One father-coach was handed a stacked deck. "I realized that in the draft we had gotten three really strong lacrosse players, but we were only supposed to get two." A lot of fathers might have kept the extra player to beef up the team. Not this dad. Instead he gave the player back. Way to lead your team to real victory.

Another dad pulled his son back to teach him humility and compassion. Eight-year-old Karl had scored four goals in the first fifteen minutes of the soccer game. The other team, which hadn't won a game all season, looked defeated already. So Karl's dad, who was coaching, benched him. Karl cried, begging to be put back in the game. His dad was patient, but he held the line. "I know you want to play, Karl, but these kids haven't scored a single goal, and you have four. Let these kids have a chance. Sometimes doing the right thing doesn't feel good, but it's still right."

Doing the right thing has enormous value. A sixth-grade teacher was frustrated that her students were cheating and wanted to help them make moral choices. She told them that if she made a grading mistake in their favor and they pointed it out—even though it would lower their grade—the whole class would get a reward. Self-reporting spiked, and cheating dropped. The kids got a pizza party, but, most of all, they learned the importance of honesty.

"The word character *is from the old French word* caractere *and means imprint on the soul."*

—Michael Bernard Beckwith, spiritual leader and author

What do you want to imprint on your child's soul? When parents think about a child's future, they dream of their child becoming a really good person. Teach your children about character. That's the best place to invest your attention. Talk to your kids about ethical choices and what you truly value. Teach them that good choices domino. Give your kids an ethical barometer, a soul compass. Hardwire character into children's formation of self.

It was the last game of the Texas high school basketball season. The coach decided that in the last few minutes, no matter the score, he would play his team manager, a boy with developmental disabilities who adored basketball. Teammates fed Mitchell the ball, but he missed repeated attempts at baskets. When he knocked the ball out of bounds with ten seconds left, one of his opponents, Jonathon, was supposed to throw it in to a teammate.

Instead Jonathon got Mitchell's attention and threw him the ball. Mitchell scored. The crowd went crazy. Mitchell's accomplishment electrified them. But Jonathon's was just as laudable. His spirit of compassion and kindness captured the crowd—and the country when the video went viral. A CBS reporter asked why Jonathon had thrown the ball to Mitchell. "I was raised to treat others how you want to be treated," he responded. It was just that simple. And just that big.

The reporter captured the magnitude of the moment, and the lesson for life: "It was not the game-winning shot. . . . But Jonathon's assist and Mitchell's basket did change the outcome decidedly. Play any game with this much sportsmanship and both teams win."

Shrink Notes

Prada Kids

1. Parenting is not a project—it is a relationship. We are spending too much time on the wrong stuff.
2. Have perspective. Our goal is to raise kind and moral kids. Our happiness ultimately stems from our connections to people.
3. Our myopic focus on "success" prevents us from seeing who our children really are and erodes our connection to them.
4. We need to let go of the notion that self-esteem comes from athletic wins and perfect grades. Loosen up on the external résumé. There is no such thing as a Prada kid.
5. Children need your love, not intrusion, interference, or micromanaging. We are supposed to embody balance, not fuel anxiety.
6. Easing your own anxiety will pay bigger dividends than fads like flash cards or music in utero.
7. When we've pushed our kids so hard they turn to stimulants to study, we have gone way too far. Stimulants are for ADHD, not for academic edge.
8. Obsessing about performance makes love feel conditional. Let your children know you will love them no matter the score of the game or the college they attend.
9. Cheer from the bleachers. Don't berate or coach.
10. Model and highlight good behavior and actions that show character. Make being a good person the most important achievement.

CHAPTER SEVEN

Moderating Media

> In barely one generation, we've moved from exulting in time-saving devices that have so expanded our lives to trying to get away from them—often in order to make much more time. The more ways we have to connect, the more many of us seem desperate to unplug.
>
> —Pico Iyer, author and essayist

Rita, a college professor in Chicago, was trying to find a little peace after a hectic semester of teaching and competing for her students' attention against a barrage of texts and e-mails. So she went to a Buddhist retreat. They breathed, they chanted, they meditated. After a particularly deep meditation, Rita gently opened her eyes. Her gaze drifted to a young monk, a four-year-old boy in an orange robe, his shaved head bent and bathed in sunlight. She was surprised to see such a young boy praying so intently. Except, he wasn't. He was playing a Game Boy.

Technology is everywhere and has brought us so many

advantages. We can connect with others around the world with speed and efficiency we never could have imagined. Advancements in education, medicine, business, and the arts have been extraordinary.

But progress can have a shadow side, and one of our jobs as parents is to be thoughtful about how we incorporate technology into our children's lives.

It's tough, because new gadgets and apps keep exploding onto the scene in rapid succession. We just add another electronic device to our lives or use a new app or social media outlet without giving much thought to its effect. But electronic devices are meant to be tools, not a way of life. Parents really should take time to think through how media and electronics are altering the landscape of childhood.

One mom who has children ten years apart feels the difference in the last decade. "I used to argue with my older son about playing Mario Kart. That battle was limited to home. But with the introduction of games on the iPhone, my fights with his younger siblings seem to know no end."

Media is ubiquitous. *National Geographic Kids* reports that, laid end to end, all the iPhones and iPads sold in one year would stretch halfway around the world.

And the portability of electronics is truly a parenting game changer. Back in the day you couldn't lug your boulder-size, antenna-attached, plug-in TV—much less wall-based telephone—out to dinner. Now, with smartphones and tablets, all of humankind seems mesmerized by devices everywhere you go. There is even an iPotty that lets toddlers play video games to take the pressure off going to the bathroom. Now we have to iPoop?

This electronic train is racing full speed ahead. We are living like real-life Jetsons without taking stock of its effect on the quality of our children's lives. Meanwhile, more parents are letting their kids use apps without knowing how it affects child or brain development. Too many of us are assuming it is harmless and justifying kid's media use for fear our children are falling behind in a competitive electronic world.

But kids will catch up on computer skills in a nanosecond. It's much harder to play catch-up on the emotional and social skills that children can develop only by interacting with other human beings. Learning to negotiate shared toys in the sandbox is more important at this age than learning to protect a virtual garden from zombies.

PARENTING VERSUS PACIFYING

I was at the post office and saw an exuberant three-year-old girl with her mom. The girl began asking her mother questions, trying to understand how post offices work. Her mother answered a few times, then continued addressing her packages. The daughter's questions persisted. Her mom grew impatient and snapped. The little girl started to cry. Rather than comfort her and apologize, the mom took out her cell phone and said, "Here, play Angry Birds." The girl immediately quieted. I was struck by how reflexively this mother used the game to calm her daughter, ignoring the feelings her daughter needed to work through. I was even more dismayed that it worked.

One of our biggest roles as parents is being an emotion coach. The little girl was curious. She got frustrated when

Mom didn't pay attention. Mom had an opportunity to model patience and teach her daughter how to delay gratification; instead she just pacified her. Then, once the girl cried, Mom missed the chance to reconnect with her daughter and help her understand her feelings. Instead she numbed them. And it worked. The game hypnotized the little girl, as if a wand were waved in front of her face. She was completely absorbed in the sight of a bird with a bad attitude being slung at a green pig.

The psychological implications of using a game in place of mothering are staggering. I spend so much time working to help my patients access the feelings they've ignored or medicated with excessive work, alcohol, food, and so forth. These are such tough habits to break. When we numb our children's feelings with the "convenient" distraction of electronics instead of teaching them to recognize and deal with their emotions, we are setting them up to follow this same impulse in adulthood. I beg you to resist the easy out and work through those moments.

No electronic device can ever substitute for human interaction. Electronics don't build emotional skills. Being with other people does. Our brains are wired for bonding. Remember, you're trying to grow a more resilient brain and foster mental health. We don't even notice how reflexive it's become to use the ever-present smartphone as a parenting crutch. I am not talking about electronics as an occasional babysitter. Many parents fall back on electronics when they need a break. Tablets on airplanes are nothing short of lifesavers. Even a wonderful therapist, who specializes in parent-child attachment, told me: "Look, I have two young kids, and I turn on the TV so that I can make dinner. But that is very different from using technology in place of mothering."

I was at Target and saw a little girl with her mom. The daughter, who looked around twenty months old, was fussing in the cart. The mom grabbed her cell phone to placate her. It worked for a brief moment, but the daughter did not have the coordination to hold the phone and play the game at the same time. The phone kept dropping on the floor. The mom looked at me with pride: "I have the best mom invention. Target should install iPads in the grocery carts—how's that for a great parenting idea?"

Boy, did she have the wrong audience.

Our brains are wired for human interaction. We are not emotionless computers. When big feelings are worked through, rather than avoided, a child learns to feel at home with herself. Over time she internalizes a nurturing and attuned parent, and that is how she ultimately learns to self-soothe.

Computers can't teach that. They can only placate.

Five-year-old Haley was having problems with separation anxiety and did not want her mother to leave her at a playdate. Haley constantly looked up from the board game she was playing with her friend to make sure her mom was staying put.

"I have to run errands, honey, and I will be back," her mother said. Haley became visibly anxious as her mom began to make her way to the door. "I have a great idea, honey. I'll get the iPad out of our car, and you guys can play games."

"Stay, Mommy," Haley pleaded with tears in her eyes.

Moments later, her mom was back and plopped the iPad

down in front of her. Haley immediately abandoned her board game—and her friend—and began swiping away. She became engrossed, and her mom snuck out. Oh, boy. Where did Haley's feelings go? If you don't work through separation anxiety, it doesn't miraculously vanish. It just keeps coming back.

Consider the big picture. When Haley's five, she might have a hard time navigating the first day of kindergarten. That's perfectly normal and a good opportunity to learn to work through separation fears. But if she doesn't learn to walk through her discomfort, it will keep circling back. Then when she's twenty-five, she might unconsciously cling to men, who might in turn run for the hills, perpetuating the separation-anxiety cycle. Don't you want to help her deal with it at five so she doesn't continue to struggle with it at twenty-five, thirty-five, and forty-five?

VIRTUAL ADDICTION

After swimming with his buddies in a highly chlorinated pool, eleven-year-old Jake asked his mom, Sophie, if he could use his allotted two hours of tech time to play the Xbox. When Sophie told him that it was time to stop, Jake started bawling. Sophie was used to the five-more-minutes plea, but this was decidedly different.

"What's wrong?" Sophie asked.

"My eyes have been stinging so badly, and they're blurry," Jake said, sobbing.

"Why didn't you tell me, honey?"

"Because I knew you would tell me to stop playing Xbox."

Jake's willingness to withstand burning eyes and blurry

vision would set off any mom's alarm bells. But then again, most video games are designed to be addictive.

"When we think of addiction, we usually associate it with alcoholism or drug abuse," Dr. Gary Small, author of *iBrain*, told me. "During a game, dopamine is released into the player's brain, causing intense pleasure." In that way, electronics are "just as addictive and potentially destructive."

No wonder technology detox centers are springing up around the world.

"I think video games are like candy. Parents know it's not good for kids; with candy they say no, but with video games they get confused. They shouldn't."

—Molly, twelve

When you call kids to dinner, there is a qualitative difference between a kid who has been running outside versus one who has been playing a video game. While both kids may ask for a few more minutes, the video player often seems much more anxious. His need to keep playing appears compulsive.

"I never told you this, but when I was young, video games got me all keyed up. I couldn't go to sleep for at least an hour after playing," one college senior confessed to his mom.

Kids actually can lose sleep over video games. Research shows a 22 percent decrease in melatonin, the chemical that helps you sleep, in people who use bright screens in the hours before bed.

Bright screens can even distract you from daylight.

Consider this scenario. The sun shone on a blanket of powdered snow covering a Utah mountain. As I rode the chairlift with a teenage boy, I marveled, "What an ideal ski day."

"Yeah, sure is," the boy replied.

"I was watching you ski down the last run. You are a great skier."

"Thanks."

"Do you love skiing?" I asked.

"Yes, but I can't wait for my dad to say we're done for the day so we can head back to the condo so I can play video games."

Wow, I did not see that coming. I was struck by the glorious day and the thrill of the mountain. Yet, for him, nothing beat the rush of a video game.

"My kids would rather play video games than do just about anything!"

—Universal lament of parents

While kids think they are just indulging harmless fantasy, the brain and body tell a different story. The brain does not distinguish between real life and virtual life. When you are mimicking outmaneuvering supervillains or beating Kobe Bryant to a slam dunk, your body will feel like it's actually happening. Your heart races, your breath gets short and shallow. To your nervous system, the virtual world is quite real.

Because your body thinks you are in an urgent situation, it automatically secretes cortisol. Your more primitive brain, the amygdala, lights up at the expense of the frontal cortex, where critical thinking and judgment reside. Do you really want your children's thoughtful brain continually hijacked by their primitive fight-or-flight brain?

It is difficult for research to keep up with the tech explosion. But what we do know suggests we should be careful. We know the brain evolves to accommodate its environment, and it seems as if games are already changing kids' wiring.

Michael Rich, a Harvard pediatrician and director of the Center on Media and Child Health, told the *New York Times*: "Their brains are rewarded not for staying on task but for jumping to the next thing. The worry is we're raising a generation of kids . . . whose brains are going to be wired differently."

Everything today seems to be in a short sound bite, a monosyllabic text, or a YouTube story told in one minute. You can't even look up a word in an online dictionary without a video ad screaming for your attention. Today's environment is programmed for distraction and consumerism, with text messages and e-mails pinging and compelling you to look. All that stimulation is affecting the ability to concentrate and be patient.

Teachers sure feel it.

"Today I have to design my lessons to keep my students engaged. I can no longer do a forty-five-minute lesson, only fifteen-minute ones."

—Midwestern teacher

Teachers have to take breaks more frequently and shift topics more often to keep attention from wandering. Even then students are distracted easily.

"I used to be able to walk into a classroom where kids were reading silently and nobody would know I was there. Now I walk in and kids' heads pop up before I have stepped both feet in the room."

—Longtime principal

If children don't learn to concentrate when they are young, they won't miraculously acquire focus later in life. But, today, it seems the only thing that can hold a kid's attention is an electronic device.

PLUG IN, TUNE OUT

The beach restaurant buzzed with activity. Against a background of clinking glasses and lively music, people shared food, stories, and laughter. Adults, anyway. I glanced down to the teenage end of the table. Every head was bent. No talking, no eye contact. Just six heads hunched over furious fingers tapping out no-doubt profound thoughts. Like " 'sup." And "L8r."

Unfortunately, this asocial scene is becoming all too common. Adolescents need to be practicing social skills like eye contact, reading facial expressions, discerning inflection. Instead they are lost in their own world, erecting a virtual wall between them and the people around them. It's rude, but worse yet, it's isolating.

And it's not just the kids who are immersed in their gadgets. It is common today to see a family of five around a table, all staring at their cell phones or game devices, instead of interacting with one another. This modern twist on family night out defeats its original purpose: togetherness. Why should the kids check in when their parents are already checked out?

The therapist Debra Green, who specializes in attachment, warns that distraction around children is emotionally risky: "We need to be present and responsive for attachment to form, and if our heads are buried, I worry about how it affects bonding."

Bonding, as I've said, is essential to social and emotional development. A child feels safe and connected when his primary caregiver is warm, responsive, and available. But today parents too often respond more urgently to their cell phones than to their children.

Think of how annoying the constant interruptions and distractions are to us adults. Now imagine being a kid, fully enthusiastic and craving his parent's undivided attention. No one, especially a child, wants to play second fiddle to a text message.

Charlotte, six, grew impatient watching her dad broker deals at the Thanksgiving table. So she went in the other room to make a call. To him. "Dad, how's the turkey?"

"Instead of greeting our kids when they get in the car, we are talking on the cell phone. . . . Do not answer the phone; answer the call of your child to feel valued, loved, and important."

—Beth Ekre, North Dakota Teacher of the Year

In other words, don't trade precious moments for digital ones.

I was watching a toddler discover her world at a café. She

was exploring and using language to make connections. She pointed up. "Tree. Tree. Trees look like broccoli!"

Her mother could barely tear herself away from her texting long enough to mumble, "Uh, yes, honey." The child kept talking joyfully, then, when that didn't grab her mom's attention, she covered her eyes and yelled, "BOO!"

I was so relieved when the mom looked up and said, "Oh, you want to play peekaboo?" I thought she was going to unglue her face from her phone and interact with her daughter. My heart dropped when the mom pulled out a tablet and said, "Here, play peekaboo." She handed the daughter the tablet, but the toddler pushed it away. The girl was looking out at the world, taking in three real-life dimensions, but her mom wanted her head down, focused on a flat screen. The little girl just wanted her mom to share in her delight. The mom wanted to pawn her off on electronic peekaboo.

Why would we want to replace ourselves with inanimate objects? Worse still, why would we want to hook our young kids on technology that already frustrates us in teenagers and adults?

But people seem to. One mom was thrilled that the computer could read books to her four-year-old son. "Sometimes I just get too tired and busy at night to read, so I let the computer read for me."

Yikes! Bedtime routines share more than stories. Snuggling together to read shares warmth—and shares you. Savor that precious bonding time.

A computer can never replace real intimacy—not for a child at bedtime nor for teens seeking connections online.

THE ANTISOCIAL NETWORK

At a coffeehouse I heard a teenage girl lament, "I lost seven followers today." A psychiatrist could have a field day with that statement. Teenagers, who already are so self-conscious, now are valuing themselves based on the rise and fall of followers, many of whom they probably don't even know. No matter how much Twitter, Facebook, and the like feed an alarming new appetite for mass approval, true self-esteem isn't what a bunch of followers think of you, it's what you think of yourself. Having more followers might give you a boost, but that good feeling is fleeting and needs constant reinforcement.

One high school sophomore showed me just how much strategy is required to get the ego massage teens are looking for.

"I wait to post my Facebook pictures until Friday at five, as all of my friends will be home after school, and that way I can get the most 'likes.' "

"What are you posting?" I asked, feeling my age.

"My picture," she replied, laughing at my digital naïveté.

It's not like she was sharing ideas or inspired quotes. She was sharing glamour shots. She showed me her friends' responses: *You are so pretty. Stunning. Love. Love. Perfection. Gorgeous. Love. Love. A real beauty.*

"I feel good," she told me. "I guess I feel valued when my friends make comments like that."

As a therapist, I knew what this girl was really looking for—to feel cherished and adored. She needed a parent to offer perspective, to help her realize that her true value doesn't rise and fall with Facebook "likes" or appreciation of her appearance.

"Kids today go out looking for photo ops. They want to look cool. They are less concerned about having a good time and more concerned about looking like they are having a good time."

—Graham, college junior

In other words, they are so busy documenting moments that they aren't living in them. Spending time creating an online image of a life is taking away from living a real one. Constantly posting and Photoshopping pictures of yourself fuels self-consciousness, not to mention takes self-involvement to a whole new level. And that's where parents need to come in. Parents have to encourage kids to lift their faces from their screens and look into real life. Instead of campaigning for virtual strokes, parents need to help teens realize that they will find life much richer by building a handful of real, caring friendships.

It is hard to form true friendships, though, if you do not know how to interact socially. Emotional and social skills have great predictive value for success, Daniel Goleman noted in his landmark book *Emotional Intelligence*. EQ can matter more than IQ, he said. There is a critical window for developing these skills, while the brain is forming and most malleable, from infancy to college. Let's make sure our kids build those skills and are able to understand social and emotional nuances such as facial expression and tone instead of only clipped code language from a backlit screen. It's so challenging today.

"On numerous occasions, I have stood on the sidelines watching my two daughters attempting to deal with sticky

situations via text message. At times, I have proposed to them, 'Just pick up the phone; wouldn't that be less complicated?' The answer is always 'NO,' along with an annoyed face that I don't believe can be effectively represented by any emoticon."

—Fran Lasker, psychotherapist

Communication is sophisticated. Even adults struggle with its subtleties. Kids need to practice these skills, and the opportunities to do so are harder to come by nowadays.

"When I grew up, there was no cable. TV had the news and a few programs. There were no DVDs, no Netflix, no computers or e-mails or text. We had nothing to do but to actually talk and be with each other. I am thankful for that."

—Educator

Potential Side Effects of Tech

Decreases time playing outside	Increases sedentary behavior and obesity
Decreases time building social skills	Increases isolation and loneliness
Decreases sleep	Increases irritability
Decreases empathy	Increases desensitization
Decreases attention/memory	Increases byte-size thinking
Decreases academic performance	Increases addictive tendencies

---

BE THE CONTENT POLICE

I walked in to the movie *The Hunger Games*, having never read the book. I had not even seen a review of the movie and did not know what it was about. I sat down behind a father with his young son. They were eating candy and joking before the movie started. The boy dropped his box of Junior Mints, and I reached under the seat to give it back.

"How old are you?" I asked.

"Seven," he answered with a smile.

As the movie began, I quickly realized that the plot was about teenagers killing each other in the woods. Only one was to survive. My heart sank. So we—including that seven-year-old boy in front of me—were going to watch children hunt and stab each other for two hours and twenty minutes.

Squirming in my seat, I could not stop thinking about that little guy. The disturbing images of kids beating other kids to death were haunting enough for me. I could not imagine how terrifying they were for a child still struggling to differentiate truth from fiction. I am sure that the more sophisticated themes of the movie were lost on this young boy, but I am equally certain that the brutal images were not.

The lights came on, and his sad and scared face shook me. As they stood up, the boy was clinging to his father. And he was not the only kid in the crowd. I thought to myself, Why? Why expose young lives to excessive violence? Why implant these violent images in young psyches? I wondered about the nightmares these children would have.

It's so important for parents to protect children. We may tell ourselves "it's only a movie," but shielding our kids still matters. Research by the Wisconsin media expert Joanne Cantor, PhD, shows that "fears induced by exposure to films and TV can be remarkably persistent and hard to end."

It's been forty years since *Jaws* came out, and some people still don't think it's safe to go back in the water. Since then, increasingly sophisticated visual effects have only made the images that much more real, and that much more scary.

Even when you try to block some images, others manage to sneak past you.

"I had to literally cover my six-year-old's eyes when commercials came on during the Olympics. It makes me so angry that disturbing trailers for R-rated movies are intruding on everything. Is there no such thing as a family show anymore?"

—Distressed mom

TV news is equally unsettling. One mom wanted to make sure her kids didn't see the coverage of a school shooting. She even taped the football game her son wanted to watch so he wouldn't see news bulletins during commercials. Yet all that caution wasn't enough. Almost as soon as the game started, a ticker scrolled at the bottom listing all the kids who had died in the tragedy. And the mom was forced to explain to her child that nine-year-olds like him are sometimes killed. No matter how she couched it, she knew her son would be frightened.

The risk of accidental exposure is so high these days. And seeing constant violence is damaging to children's emotional health. Think how hopeless you feel when watching reports of senseless violence. Hopelessness and helplessness ar symptoms of depression—not something we want to engender in our children. We want to raise hopeful, compassionate people. But chronic exposure to tragedy can dim compassion, which has frightening implications.

According to a 2007 letter in the journal *Pediatrics*, the Center on Media and Child Health studied "956 scientific articles that provide nearly unanimous evidence that exposure to media violence contributes to elevated fear and anxiety, sleep disturbances, desensitization to human suffering, and an increase in aggressive thoughts and behaviors."

We're trying to raise kind, caring, optimistic kids. So we have to monitor what they're watching—from cynicism to violence to sexuality.

> *"Children do not have the mental faculties to process a lot of information . . . especially information about issues and things far beyond their scope of reference. Too much information does not 'prepare' a child for a complicated world; it paralyzes them."*
>
> —Kim John Payne, *Simplicity Parenting*

> *"In this digital age . . . Internet porn is almost impossible to avoid. Kids are curious, and 'porn' is now the fifth most popular Internet search term for kids age six and up."*
>
> —James P. Steyer, *Talking Back to Facebook*

six are still waiting for the tooth fairy. They are not
ysically, or emotionally equipped to handle the
f what they are seeing.

We parents should safeguard and nurture childhood's innocence, which is already so precious and fleeting. We can't rely on the entertainment industry to do it for us. One Hollywood mogul described his entirely different standards for his business and his kids: "I am a dad and I don't rely on the ratings for kids' shows. We [in the industry] lobby to get the rating that will give us the largest audience and make us the most money. We are not lobbying for what is really appropriate for kids."

So we must be our children's guardians in these formative years.

GATEKEEPERS

Shielding our kids from the intrusion of unwanted ideas and images is so much easier when they're tiny. That's when we have the most control and can limit the quantity and content of what they see. The longer you can put off the introduction of electronics, the better you can protect a kid's innocence and prolong the wonder of childhood. And that is so worth protecting!

As you slowly introduce media, make sure the proportions are right. Find programs that inspire. Accentuate the positive and try to minimize the negative.

For instance, one of Oprah Winfrey's last episodes highlighted the scholarships she generously gave to 415 men who attended Morehouse College. With video images of run-down communities in the background, one man after another described how Oprah's gift had given him the opportunity to change his life. Now they all are educated men, committed to paying their good fortune forward. As Oprah was serenaded by the lyrics "Because we knew you, we have been changed for good," the scholarship recipients streamed into the dark stadium, their grown faces lit only by the candles in their hands.

That episode made people cry. It touched them. It made them want to do good themselves. Seeing kindness is good for the body, mind, and soul. We have medical proof. A Harvard study documented this "Mother Teresa Effect." When students watched a video of Mother Teresa's compassionate acts, their immune function increased. Doing and even just watching good deeds also increased serotonin levels, which improve mood and calmness. Acts of kindness and compassion are organic Prozac.

So make sure you know what type of media your kids are ingesting. And make sure, with all the video candy in their digital diet, that you are feeding them positive messages, too. Teach them to use common sense, think about their values, and develop judgment to make good choices. Talk about what is appropriate and what is not.

"The good news is that this kind of parental involvement has a positive effect. Research shows that it can make a huge difference in the amount of media that kids consume. That's important, because studies have shown that kids who spend less time with media have far better grades in school and higher levels of personal contentment."

—James P. Steyer, *Talking Back to Facebook*

Overconsumption is not the only reason for caution. Kids need to know that there is no such thing as privacy today—

and that privacy has huge value. It's almost inconceivable how far and fast information flies the minute you push send. Help your kids realize that what they think they are "just sharing with a friend" is going to exist forever digitally and can be seen by everyone. Even a "private" text can be forwarded around the world in a second.

You have to teach them to ask themselves: Would I be comfortable with this post or picture going viral? What if my parents or teachers saw it? Will I still be comfortable when a job interviewer stumbles on it in five years?

It is important to make young people practice this kind of thinking. The frontal lobe of the brain, where judgment and discernment reside, is still developing into their twenties. Kids and teens need help thinking through the risks and rewards of their actions. Talk it out, help them practice and grow these skills, then calmly offer guidance if you see them veering off course.

It's so easy to overreact—"You posted *what*?"—but try not to. The key to getting them to edit themselves responsibly is to keep the conversation flowing, and let them know that you are an available resource, not a harsh judge, when they have questions.

Laying out the rules in writing is a great way to teach kids responsibility. This really works when you are extending them privileges. Have a contract before you hand them a cell phone or car keys. Clearly laying out expectations lets them know what they have to do to keep their privileges, and what behavior puts them at risk for losing them.

A mom I know wrote a cell phone agreement for her kids, and a dad wrote up a driving contract for his son. Both are at the end of this chapter as guidance for when you need to spell out responsibilities.

UNPLUG

Of course, our best strategy for getting young people to manage their digital diet is to watch our own. Most parents are not even conscious of how much time they themselves are using electronics.

When one boy got sick of his dad telling him he couldn't play on the Wii all day, he shot back: "Have you seen yourself, Dad? You have trouble finishing a sentence without looking down at your phone."

Luckily the dad felt the effect of his son's words. He and his son devised a plan. Every time the dad looked at his phone in the car or at dinner, his son got a dollar to donate to the charity of his choice. As the dollar bills piled up, Dad started to see the light.

"I really was surprised by how my texting was interfering with my relationships at home. I wasn't even really aware of it. When my son pointed out what I was doing, I knew it was time to change. . . . My son felt happier and—after my initial anxiety died down—so did I."

Taking a digital reprieve is restorative.

"My father had a very busy career, but when he came home, he was home. I, too, have a demanding job, but when I get home from work, I answer e-mails and return calls. My wife pointed out to me that even at home I was still at work. I knew that she was right. I stopped checking e-mails until

after my kids went to bed. We now have family dinners and nights free of distractions. I like myself more as a dad."

—Untethered father

Once you learn to manage your own online impulses, you can teach your kids to manage theirs.

One mother, tired of seeing her teenage daughter and friends buried on their individual phones, made a new rule: "When they enter my house, my kids' friends know that they take off their shoes and leave them by the front door, and they take out their phones and put them in the basket next to their shoes. One prevents dirt, the other fosters friendship."

Turning off screens can be a spiritual reboot for the whole family.

"I was so fed up with the begging for TV and video games," one mom said. "I was always fighting against screens' addictive pull. I had a dream that I was cutting all of the cords in my house, and when I woke up . . . I decided to pull the plug. I declared one week of no TV or computer. My preteen kids said things like 'You can't be serious' and 'What will we do for that week?' "

The chorus of complaints only strengthened her resolve to disconnect. "I was most surprised how quickly shutting off electronics reset the balance in my house. I also noticed that without screens I was more present myself."

Another mom chose to ban electronics for a week for adults and kids alike.

"The whole feeling of my home changed. Everything seemed more peaceful. The constant and annoying TV noise was silenced. The board games that languished on the shelf—

some still in shrink-wrap—were finally dusted off. My kids were making forts and inventing games and really playing together."

These families serve as a reminder that there are many wonderful ways to spend time that do not involve electronic screens. Hours logged in front of screens are hours we miss being together. Just as the dying man won't look back fondly on all of the hours he worked, childhood's sweetest memories will not be logged in front of video games.

"If I had my life to live over . . . I would have cried and laughed less while watching television and more while watching life."

—Erma Bombeck

Shrink Notes

Moderating Media

1. Model a lack of digital distraction yourself. Check in; don't check out.
2. Electronics are not pacifiers. When kids are upset, teach them to work through their feelings.
3. Regulate media so it doesn't steal childhood. Monitor and have rules for young kids; teach older ones to monitor themselves.
4. Electronics, games, and videos are addictive. Teach moderation.
5. The body doesn't distinguish between real life and virtual life. All stress feels real.
6. You don't want your kids desensitized to gratuitous violence or to shut down. You want to build empathy and compassion into their growing brains.
7. Negative imagery is enduring and toxic for developing psyches.
8. Positive images inspire good feelings and good neurochemistry.
9. Check out CommonSenseMedia.org for a great parent guide to media.
10. Make sure you have more real moments than digital ones.

PHONE AGREEMENT

Dear Beth:

Now that you are entering seventh grade, we are happy to give you a smartphone to use. Having a phone is fun and useful, but also a privilege. You will have the responsibility of honoring the rules below as a condition of enjoying the phone. You have always been very responsible, and we're confident that you'll continue to earn our trust.

1. The phone is owned by us, and we have the right to restrict its use, monitor it, or take it away at any time.
2. The phone is to be used to connect and communicate with your friends and family, and not for any inappropriate behavior.
3. The phone will never be used to bully, intimidate, or make hurtful comments about other people, even if the messages aren't being sent to them. Words are powerful. Use them for good.
4. You will honor all rules outside the house about appropriate phone use. For example, at school, you will use the phone only at designated times and places that the school allows. If you're caught texting in a classroom, for example, we will take the phone away.
5. The phone will never be allowed at mealtime. That is our time to connect and unplug. This applies whether eating at home or out.

6. The phone should be in the off position when you are studying. Constant texting is a distraction that will negatively affect your study habits.
7. Anything you send over the phone may end up in the public domain. So never send ANYTHING that you wouldn't want your parents or teachers to see. Even if an app deletes a photo, it can and might be saved.
8. Use your good judgment. Never send inappropriate or risqué photos of yourself. They may stay on the Internet forever. That's a long time.
9. Remember that communicating via smartphone shouldn't interfere with life. Try to focus on what's happening around you, rather than sharing the experience via text, e-mail, or social media.

____

Beth

____

Parent(s)

DRIVING CONTRACT

This contract is between Billy, a minor child, and his parents, _______________ ("Parents"). Parents join Billy in his excitement at reaching this milestone. Because both parties agree that driving is a privilege and a huge responsibility, they have agreed to abide by the terms of this contract. Parents have trust in Billy and confidence that he will meet the following terms and conditions:

1. The [insert model/year of vehicle] ("Car") is owned by parents, and all rights associated with ownership shall be theirs, including but not limited to the right to sell the vehicle.
2. Billy cannot modify the car in any manner without the express approval of parents, and it is noted that such approval shall not be readily forthcoming. This shall include, but not be limited to, modifying the appearance of the vehicle, changing the sound system, or any modifications to the performance of the vehicle.
3. Billy shall not have the right to ever sell, lease, lend, or trade in the car without the express written approval of parents. He shall never lend the car to a friend without the express prior approval of parents. The value of this car shall not be his to ultimately trade in.
4. Billy agrees to pay for gasoline used for the car.
5. Billy agrees to be responsible for following the maintenance schedule recommended by the manufacturer.

6. As owner, parents shall have the right to use the car at any time, including but not limited to lending it to their friends from time to time.
7. Parents shall have the right to rescind or restrict Billy's use of the car at any time, for any reason whatsoever.
8. Parents shall initially pay for insurance (this policy is subject to future modification). However, Billy agrees to pay for 100 percent of any insurance increase that is caused by a ticket or accident.
9. If Billy receives a moving violation, he shall lose for 60 calendar days the privilege of driving the car. Parents may reduce this penalty if they deem, in their sole judgment, that citation was the result of inexperience rather than poor driving behavior. Speeding tickets, going through red lights, or rolling through stop signs shall be automatically deemed to fall into the poor driving behavior category.
10. If Billy receives a citation for reckless driving that is upheld by a judge, he shall forfeit for 1 year his right to drive the car. Reckless driving is a designation by the police department for a very serious violation, such as excessive speeding (going 75 mph in a 35 mph zone, for example). It is defined as "operation of an automobile in a dangerous manner under the circumstances, including speeding, cutting in and out of traffic, failing to yield to other vehicles, and other negligent acts. It is a misdemeanor crime." There will be zero tolerance for reckless driving.

11. There will be zero tolerance for drinking and driving. If Billy drinks even a trace of alcohol and gets behind the wheel, he shall forfeit for 6 months the right to drive the vehicle.
12. If Billy receives a DUI (defined as being at the adult legal threshold for being drunk as opposed to having a trace amount of alcohol in his system) which is upheld by a judge, he shall indefinitely forfeit his right to drive, and this will likely lead to the sale of the vehicle.
13. Billy agrees that the music system in the car will remain off until parents deem him ready to manage it.
14. Billy agrees to abide by all Department of Motor Vehicles laws that pertain specifically to 16-year-old drivers. If he breaks curfew or drives with another minor in the car (as defined by DMV), his privilege to drive the car shall be rescinded for 30 calendar days, whether or not he is cited for such violation. The only exception shall be for cases where prior approval is granted by parents.
15. Billy agrees to abide by new laws forbidding 16-year-old drivers from using cell phones while driving, even if hands-free (with a bona fide emergency being the only exception). If Billy violates this law, even if not cited by the police, he shall lose for 30 calendar days his privilege of driving the car. For example, if parents call his cell phone and he answers while driving, then he is in violation of applicable laws and will lose driving privileges per above. A second violation will lead to loss of driving privileges for 90 calendar days. Sending or reading text messages while driving will cause the loss of driving privilege for

90 days. This also applies when at red lights or stopped in traffic. Parents shall have the right to periodically check cell phone records to see if there is any cell phone activity during periods of driving. Until the following rule is waived by parents, the cell phone must be in off position (airplane mode) at all times that the vehicle is turned on. There will be zero tolerance for driving and using the cell phone.

16. Billy acknowledges that driving as a minor is a privilege that carries with it important obligations to other drivers as well as to himself. Billy agrees to make his best effort to drive carefully, courteously, calmly, and with respect for other drivers, and to make his best effort to be a safe and responsible driver.

Agreed to and Accepted:

By:

____

Minor Date

By:

____

Parent Date

CHAPTER EIGHT

Life Is Remembered in the Pauses

We do too much and savor too little. We mistake activity for happiness, and so we stuff our children's days with activities, and their heads with information, when we ought to be feeding their souls instead.

—Katrina Kenison, *Mitten Strings for God*

Karen's three kids were always playing sports. As they grew, so did the sports schedule. It got more and more unwieldy.

"I was so stressed-out running to get each of my children to their respective fields, screaming, 'Get in the car, we are going to be late,' twenty times a day, that I started to fantasize about having a washer/dryer in my minivan. I thought, If I could just find a way to do laundry in my minivan, I could win back some time."

Now, that's some fantasy—turn the family car into a Laundromat. Karen finally threw up her hands and stopped the spin cycle.

"That was my aha moment. I started making choices to simplify. I began with making a small, doable change each day. I started cutting back on a few activities per week. We were all so much happier."

Why don't more of us make changes to simplify our schedules? Because we are so caught up in the idea of not missing any opportunity for our children. Not only are we starting early, we're packing on the activities. But more isn't better. Children need time to breathe. And so do their parents.

"I don't know when Sunday became the new Saturday. But I don't like it. I want to just be with my family at home on a Sunday."

—West Coast mother of four

Today's high-tech, fast-paced world is on a collision course with childhood. Once upon a time, we remembered the Sabbath day and kept it holy—or at least tranquil. Nowadays, even when you try to give your kids or yourself a break, you run into obstacles.

"I decided to not schedule my kids in any activities for a semester, and there were very few kids left to play with who were not on sports teams or in some other organized activity."

—East Coast mom

That's how far our frenzied pendulum has swung. Even those who don't board the Super Activity Bus feel it. Many parents recognize the madness but still adopt "if you can't beat 'em, join 'em" mentalities.

How can we bridge the distance between what we cherished most about our own childhoods and what we are giving to our kids? Remember when days and play were unhurried, unstructured, and could unfold organically, without a to-do list? Summer days at the beach, floating in the waves for hours; running with our friends in a pack around our neighborhoods; lying on our backs, staring at the sky, imagining shapes in the clouds.

Can we recapture some of that and stop all of this running around? Let's find a way to keep home and family a soft place to land, an easy place to be, a port for recharging.

EASE OFF THE SCHEDULE

"My three-year-old was mesmerized by a ladybug. Quietly crouched to the ground, she was examining it closely with wonder. I called her to get in the car, as we were going to be late for her toddler gym class. She was so engaged with the ladybug that she did not even hear me. So I swooped down, grabbed her, strapped her into her car seat, and shoved a toy in her lap. Tears started rolling down her face.

"At that moment, lightning struck. I thought, What am I doing to her? Why am I pulling her away from a ladybug to rush her to a synthetic gym with a whole bunch of three-year-olds who would also rather be playing with bugs?"

—Mom who found peace in simplicity

Watching a ladybug is like a meditation. It is a way of feeling connected, an experience of oneness with nature, a sense of peace. Of course this little tyke found it jarring to be yanked away.

Children need space and time to feel their spirit. We used to honor childhood's natural rhythm. But these days, frenzy rules.

"I spend a lot of time after work racing my kids from one activity to the next. We're lucky if we have time to hit the drive-through. One day my guilt got the best of me and I decided that I was going to slow down the pace in our house and cook a really good homemade meal. When I was done and feeling very proud, I yelled, 'Dinner!' Nobody came. They had run to the car and buckled themselves in."

—Bewildered mom

We have made activities, not family dinner, the priority. This is backward. The bonding families get over the dinner table will bring your children more security and happiness than rushing from piano lessons to baseball. Family dinner is an essential ingredient to a healthy child. Study after study links family dinner to a lower incidence of drug and alcohol use and lower obesity rates.

The constant hustle from activity to activity makes you feel frayed and stressed. Your anxiety goes up and your tolerance for frustration goes down. Bad enough for adults. The effect on children's brains, still under construction and so vulnerable to stress, is even greater.

"I am embarrassed to say that I had my kids overscheduled to a crazy degree. I was the Tiger Mom on steroids. I had my kids in activities seven days a week, from morning till night. My three girls were taking art classes, swimming lessons, gymnastics, studying Spanish, and going to religious school. And they were all under ten!

"My kids seemed unhappy. They were having trouble sleeping, and there was a whole lot of whining going on. One day my daughter said that she always felt too rushed and that it would be nice to have a few days a week to play with her friends or her sister or by herself."

—Hurried mom of harried kids

Wow. Mom needed to let go—and she did! She took a red pen and slashed 80 percent of the schedule. She felt free. So did her children. They were happy being kids. She returned to them what she had never intended to steal: their childhood.

LOOSEN THE REINS

On vacation in a rural town, Sandy, ten, was mesmerized by the sight of kids riding bikes in a pack. She ran into the kids again later at the ice cream store. They started having a friendly conversation. Then Sandy posed the question that she had been curious about all day.

"Where are your parents?" she asked.

"At home," one boy said with a shrug.

"You are so lucky! You can ride a bike and hang out by yourself?" she questioned.

"Yeah, sure," a couple of kids answered.

"Wow, that is so cool," Sandy said. "I am never alone."

How sad. Kids today have very few moments to themselves without a parent hovering, a babysitter monitoring, or a coach supervising. We need to step back and give them space to dream and play.

How can you discover yourself when you have no time to be with yourself? Kids learn so much when they are doing things on their own: self-reliance, self-initiation, and just being at home with their own company. When children can find their way, instead of having parents direct them, they become more engaged and empowered. Kids need practice in this. But practice is hard to come by when a big person is watching your every move.

One mom got it. She told her babysitter she was there as a safety net, not as an entertainment center. Instead of finding things for the kids to do, the babysitter should relax in the other room and read magazines, letting the kids play on their own. If she heard screams or saw blood, the mom said, she should spring into action. Otherwise she should just keep reading. This smart mom recognized that kids don't need constant prompting. They need to know how to entertain themselves.

Past generations of parents gave us a lot of freedom to go out and play, as long as we were back by a certain hour. That gave us a sense of independence and an ability to go out and discover the world and figure out how far we were willing to stretch. For all its faults, benign neglect gave us room to explore.

"When I was a little girl, we would visit my grandmother, who lived near the woods in Wisconsin. I can still recall

the smell of the woods—and the feeling of being set free in nature as my sister and I played and explored. We would create little rooms in the woods. A clearing of three trees marked our living room, and a group of wildflowers represented the kitchen. We'd take rocks and build our own furniture. We would play for hours dreaming up our house in the woods."

—Chicago college professor

Freedom. Dreaming. Exploring. Wonder. This is the magic of childhood.

LET THEM PLAY

At a recent parenting lecture, a woman asked the speaker's advice: "My five-year-old just wants to do imaginary play for hours. How can I get him to stop wasting time and do something more productive?"

Was she kidding? Imaginary play is such a wonderfully rich experience for a child. Parents shouldn't squash play out of their own neuroses to create a superchild.

Like many parents, this mother was operating on the faulty notion that drilling flash cards is more educational than pretend play. Years of research prove the opposite. Robbing a kid of play undermines real development. Many studies show a correlation between early imaginative play and future creativity. And boredom is pregnant with possibilities.

Nine-year-old Caine grew weary with sitting around his dad's used-auto-parts store in East L.A. all summer. While Dad was busy working, there were no planned activities, there was no specialty camp. But there was a whole lot of free time and some empty cardboard boxes.

Caine started thinking about what those boxes could be. Soon he had transformed the cardboard into a carnival-style arcade. Caine pulled together tickets and prizes, then waited and waited for his first customer. In walked Nirvan Mullick. He was blown away by what Caine had created and plopped down two dollars for a fun pass allowing him to play all the games.

Then Nirvan told Caine and his dad that he was a filmmaker, and they let him create a documentary of this young boy's adventure. Once the video hit YouTube, Caine became a national sensation, igniting kids' imaginations around the globe.

Boredom allowed Caine's creativity to take flight. And Caine proved that kids can be their own fun pass.

But too many kids, it seems, have lost that ability.

"It's really sad. For as long as I can remember, we set up a play fire station. We would leave the costumes and props out, and children historically jumped right in, being firemen, rescuing cats and putting out fires. But this year my preschoolers stared at the costumes, confused. One boy asked, 'How do we do this? What are the rules? How do you win?' I thought, Do I have to teach these kids how to play?"

—Preschool owner

"I feel like electronic games and too many lessons have

permanently changed childhood. It used to be that kids played with toys. Now if the toys don't play for the kids, they are not interested. I hope that play does not become a lost art."

—Toy store owner

With conscious effort, some parents have managed to preserve the spirit of play.

At a dinner party, while parents were talking and laughing around the table, their kids were having their own good time in another room. The children's ability to entertain themselves was remarkable. No one was whining or asking for television or video games. They were just playing. How refreshing.

Most of the kids there had attended the same preschool, which discouraged early TV or computer game use and encouraged simple toys that invited imagination. While the grown-ups entertained each other, the kids entertained themselves. They built forts, played pretend, and constructed giant creations out of blocks.

Amazing what you can unleash when you give kids room to play. Besides, they chafe under too many restrictions.

Henry, seven, grew frustrated when his mom said no to one too many of his ideas for playing with his friends.

"I wish you were more funtaneous," he moped.

Talk about a wakeup call. His mom grabbed some cans of shaving cream and told the boys to finger-paint on the windows. They stared at her in disbelief. Then they dove in. Next thing she knew, she heard giggles and squeals coming from the backyard.

The boys gleefully covered each other from head to toe in white shaving cream. They loved it.

Sometimes it is hard to loosen up. But go for it!

"I have to fight against my own instincts for everything to be neat and clean and to have my kids be 'busy' doing something. I am surprised that I struggle with this, as I really cherished the free time of my own childhood.

"One day I was making dinner and it started to pour. My kids asked if they could go outside. I have to admit, I immediately pictured wet and muddy kids dragging dirt all over my house and my dinner getting cold. Then I remembered my own childhood freedoms, and forced 'Sure! Why not? Great idea!' out of my mouth.

"They raced out the door and started jumping in puddles. My four-year-old took a running leap into an enormous mud puddle and stood up laughing.

"I was so glad that I could loosen up enough to let my kids have fun. The cold dinner and mud was a small price to pay for that invaluable memory."

—Emily, Michigan mom

Let's not sanitize the fun out of childhood. Play lets you use your imagination, which fosters creativity. When kids negotiate who gets what toy or who goes first, they learn to work out their differences. When they play pretend, they get to try on different roles (good guy, bad guy, and every guy or gal in between) and see how they fit. That teaches them what they like and don't like. It also teaches them to understand feelings.

In fact, play is such an important tool for exploring feelings that child psychiatrists use it in therapy.

Four-year-old Oliver's mother took him to counseling after Oliver lost his father in a car crash. During play sessions, his psychiatrist noted, Oliver would often cry that his pretend characters had to go to heaven too soon. By talking about the characters' deaths, the psychiatrist was able to get Oliver to open up about his own loss and begin to heal.

One time after his session, Oliver went out into the waiting room and spotted the doctor's next patient. Grabbing the young man's hands in his, Oliver said: "You are going to be OK. My dad died, too." The young man's dad hadn't actually died, but Oliver recognized that he was in pain. Through play, Oliver had learned to express and work through his feelings, giving him the capacity to identify another person's sorrow and offer comfort.

Play can be a tool for healing or a vehicle for fun. It is good for the mind, body, and spirit. Nothing is more "productive" than that.

KEEP IT SIMPLE

Elena's five-year-old daughter, Mimi, had always wanted to dress up in her princess costume and visit the Magic Kingdom castle. So Elena promised her a trip to Disneyland for her birthday.

The closer the weekend got, the more Elena began to dread it. Her husband had been doing a lot of traveling for work and was absolutely exhausted. Elena kept picturing the long, hot lines and the exorbitant expense of the day. After some second-guessing, Elena followed her instincts and told Mimi she had a different birthday idea.

"Honey, I know we promised you a trip to Disneyland today, but what if we had a princess party here instead? You, your sister, and I could all dress up as princesses, and we could dress Daddy as the prince. We could set up a whole tea party in the backyard."

Much to Elena's surprise, Mimi wasn't disappointed. She was thrilled.

"That would be so fun to have a real princess tea party!" Mimi exclaimed, jumping up and down.

As promised, Elena put on something sparkly and dressed her girls in tiaras and tutus. The sisters giggled at their dad, wearing a paper crown they had adorned with glitter.

Mimi asked her mom if all of the tea party food could be pink—after all, this was a princess party—and so they made pink smoothies, decorated their cupcakes in pink frosting, and dipped fruit into pink strawberry yogurt. It was like a special spell enveloped them as they dined like king and queens—laughing, close, happy. They had found the real Magic Kingdom in their very own backyard.

You don't have to go far or create elaborate plans to make beautiful memories. Keeping things simple makes room for magic. And simple is often just more fun.

"My son and I were invited to an old-fashioned birthday party. They played musical hula hoops, tossed water balloons, and jumped through sprinklers. The kids, who had all been to far more extravagant birthday parties, seemed to revel in this one. On the way home my son told me

that it was the best birthday party he had ever been to."

—Appreciative mom

Sometimes all you need for a party is two people.

Faye, a divorced mom, felt tired and overwhelmed. She had only two Saturdays off a month and just a few hours after work to spend with her daughter, Liza. She really wanted to take her daughter on a trip but just did not have the time or the money.

Faye decided to shake off her frustration and began thinking up ways to cherish the time they did have. Faye told Liza that in two weeks they would have a picnic on top of a mountain about a mile from where they lived. Nine-year-old Liza perked up at the idea. And the two of them jumped into the planning.

They dug out the picnic basket and put it on the kitchen counter. Then, each night for the next two weeks, they would add something to the basket: silverware and napkins, a small bud vase for a flower they might find, containers for all the food that they were going to make. One night they baked homemade muffins. The next night they put in their favorite jam. As the basket grew, so did Liza's excitement.

Picnic day finally arrived. Liza and her mom hiked up the mountain and found a shady spot for their feast. As they soaked in the lovely day, Liza looked at her mom and said, "Thank you, Mommy, for the best day of my life!"

Faye was flooded with gratitude and love. She was so thankful to be able to give that gift to her daughter. They didn't need a vacation or fancy nights out. They just needed time together to create simple moments they'd treasure always.

Even when people can splurge on extravagance, simple experiences are some of the most special.

Private-school teacher Miss Peters decided to have a snow party. Her California first graders were very excited. Miss Peters told them to bring a hat and mittens so that they would not get too cold. As they spent the week learning about seasons, they grew excited about the mysterious snow party.

Miss Peters overheard one little girl, Isabelle, tell her friend: "I went skiing in Colorado. I bet they are going to bring us snow from there."

"I bet they're going to *make* the snow!" her friend answered.

The teacher thought, Boy, are these kids going to be disappointed.

The afternoon of the snow party arrived. Miss Peters explained that first, they needed to do a little math. "We are going to learn fractions." The students groaned.

She gave them each a piece of paper and asked them to rip it down the middle.

"How much is that?" she asked.

"Half," one boy answered.

"Now tear it again. How many pieces do you see?"

"Four."

"Yes, that is one-fourth."

The exercise dragged on for a while. Just as the kids were approaching fed up, Miss Peters said, "Next, crunch up all of the paper on the desk."

Confused, they followed directions.

Then Miss Peters screamed: "Snowball fight!"

The giddy kids threw their paper at each other. Howls of

laughter seeped out of the classroom. Once they were worn-out, but still clad in hats and mittens, they all got to drink hot chocolate as they listened to a story.

Walking to the bus with little Isabelle that afternoon, the teacher asked, "What did you think of the snow party?"

Isabelle replied: "That was the most fun that I have ever had!"

Sometimes white paper and a teacher's imagination are just enough.

"If you want to see what children can do, stop giving them things."

—Norman Douglas, writer

Let's not buy into the notion that more is more. The best gift you can give your children is your time and your love. Give *you*! Reward kids not with stuff but with your presence. Stuff is the booby prize of childhood.

Even Dr. Seuss's Grinch learned that lesson when he tried—and failed—to steal Christmas by stealing presents.

"It came without ribbons! It came without tags!
"It came without packages, boxes or bags!" . . .
"Maybe Christmas," he thought, "*doesn't* come from a store.
"Maybe Christmas . . . perhaps . . . means a little bit more!"

POCKETS OF PEACE

"When I'm not enjoying parenting, it's usually because I am not in the moment. I am rushing to get somewhere or I am

thinking about all of the things I should be doing or need to get done. When I slow down and let go . . . and just allow myself to be with my children and relax and enjoy them, I have so much more fun. I get to silently witness and cherish this miracle in front of me. . . . Home is not just a place. Home is a state of being."

—Laura Carlin, author and blogger

Being in the moment often requires letting go of your to-do list and quieting the constant ruckus from the outer world. We need to find our own equilibrium so we can help our children find theirs. It helps to build space into our days for quiet moments. You get to set your home's tempo.

"I was having a hard time with my transition from work to home. I did not want to bring the stress of my job into my house, so I struggled against my urge to immediately check e-mails. I felt keyed up when I walked in the door. I knew my kids felt it, too. I needed to do something different. So I invented a dance party. Now I walk in, hug my kids, and they run to put on the music and we dance around the kitchen. I can feel the stress of work leave me, replaced by the joy on my kids' face, which melts me."

—Chicago mom

Kids absorb your energy. If you feel frazzled and frustrated, they will, too. But if you lead with a relaxed and loving energy, that's contagious as well.

One way to reset your home's rhythm is to introduce some kind of ritual or meditation. A mindful exercise in a group called Reflective Parenting asks moms and dads to sit and observe their children for five minutes. They are supposed to clear their minds of the day's distractions and watch their children play and just be present. Parents are frequently surprised at how calm and close to their children they feel in just five minutes.

Mindfulness takes practice. Even Deepak Chopra had to learn how to shed his stressed-out doctor persona to become the spiritual guru he is today. When he learned a better way, he passed it on to his kids.

"The best gift my parents ever gave me was teaching me how to meditate. I saw how much it changed their lives, and it made my brother and me want to learn. It is such a gift to be able to find that place of peace and solitude within myself."

—Malika Chopra, 2013 lecture

Science now proves meditation is good for the brain. The Wisconsin neuroscientist Richard Davidson, MD, has discovered that meditation reduces stress and inflammation, increases compassion and focus, and simply lets the body and mind work more easily.

Whether it is meditation or another avenue, find some way to schedule downtime into your children's days—just as you would soccer or piano lessons.

"I try to create pockets of peace in my house. I have small kids, so getting them to sit still is a challenge. In winter, we light a fire and stare at it quietly, which mesmerizes them.

Or we go outside and try to listen to the different sounds of nature. It feels very peaceful and close.”

—Mother of four

My dear friend says, “Environment is the third parent.” Your home environment can affect how you feel. It also affects your neurochemistry. Your brain is a living, interactive organism, impacted by its surroundings. A peaceful home creates a more peaceful brain.

Peace is not that difficult to attain, either. Clearing out the clutter—the old toys and books that your kids have outgrown, for example—creates space and the ease of order. Simple acts like turning on beautiful music or lighting a candle can change the ambiance of a home.

One mom knew she had to change things when her kids' bath time became just one more chore, complete with whining and complaining. So she reinvented it:

“One night I ran upstairs while my husband and kids were still clearing the table. I put on a CD of nature sounds. I lit a bunch of candles and dimmed the lights.”

When the kids started to protest having to take a bath, she opened the door, and the serenity of the setting washed over them. She gave them each a dropper to add a fragrant potion to their bath. The bath complaints went down the drain, as something routine became something special.

Thoughtful touches make a huge difference, whether the environment is home, work, school—even a hospital. Fortunately, the field of medicine is beginning to catch on to the healing power of a person's surroundings.

Back when I did my psychiatry residency, I spent many

days and nights in dreary inpatient psychiatric units. The walls were sterile, with no art, no music, no life. That alone was depressing and must have compounded the mental illnesses these patients already suffered. I would imagine the hospital as a truly healing space. Good smells, a peaceful color palette, nature scenes on TVs. I just knew it had to be better for patients and more conducive to recovery.

Years later, Thomas Strouse, the medical director of the UCLA neuropsychiatric hospital, described the big changes that had come from moving the hospital to a new building. The old place was dark and gloomy—narrow hallways and a few small windows made it feel closed in and claustrophobic. The new facility was thoughtfully designed to be bright and airy. Sunlight streams through big windows into large rooms and hallways, creating a sense of space. The result? Staff turnover has dropped dramatically and so has the need to put patients in four-point restraints.

What an amazing difference transforming the aesthetics of the hospital made. By bringing in natural light and spaciousness, the hospital was able to give a sense of peace to patients and staff. Bringing nature into your home can have a similar effect.

Quinn, a mother of three in Arizona, was delighted when her son, Liam, was given a butterfly garden. They sent away for caterpillar larvae, pitched a tiny tent, and spent three weeks watching the caterpillars grow, build chrysalises, and transform into butterflies.

"We prepared the tent for our expectant butterflies as a parent would a nursery," Quinn said. "We doused carnations in sugar water and lined the bottom of the tent with orange slices. The whole process, including the waiting, invited excitement and anticipation. My son and I watched with wonder for our miracle, quietly studying the slowly changing chrysalises.

"One day I heard the most exuberant scream. 'Wings! Mom! Wings!' an elated little voice called from the kitchen. We sat at the table, marveling at the birth of three butterflies."

Awe illuminated Liam's face.

"When it was time to set them free, Liam carefully and gently unzipped the tent. A colorful butterfly flew out and perched on his tiny finger."

Watching the caterpillars change into butterflies created a metamorphosis in the family. They were so grateful they had brought nature, and a peaceful rhythm, into their lives.

That peace is magnified when you can fully immerse yourself in nature.

"I make a point of spending time outdoors with my boys every weekend. Nature is the channel that connects you with your spirit. It brings forth a perpetual state of gratitude."

—Scott, earth-connected dad

On a beach in Florida, a mom and her girls were hunting for seashells amid the crashing waves, the sun warming their skin. An old man took in the reverence as the girls placed their sea treasures in baskets. He smiled at the mother and remarked, "Welcome to God's playground."

Simply following nature's powerful rhythms lets you and yours find a oneness with the earth. But today too many kids are suffering from what Richard Louv, in his book *Last Child in the Woods*, calls a "nature-deficit disorder." Their shut-in, sedentary ways are contributing to the obesity epidemic and a general listlessness. "Unlike television, nature does not steal time; it amplifies," Louv writes.

"One of my best memories of childhood came when I was in the fifth grade," a father recalled. "My dad and I decided to go for a walk and bring home a firefly. We brought a glass jar, with the holes punched in it. We headed out to a big open field and waited."

Finally, fireflies began to sparkle against the black sky.

"I can't remember how long my dad and I lay on our backs in that field. I remember the warm, humid air, and I can still recall the feeling of lying side by side, watching fireflies in silence. We walked back home, and my little brother asked to see the fireflies. We both smiled—realizing our jar was empty."

Thirty years later, his heart is still full as the memories of that night flicker on.

Shrink Notes

Life Is Remembered in the Pauses

1. Ease up on the schedule. How can kids discover themselves when they have no time to be with themselves?
2. Children need time and freedom for unstructured play. Imaginative play fosters social, emotional, and physical growth.
3. Let your kids get bored. Boredom is pregnant with possibilities.
4. Let go of the notion that they need to be "doing something productive." They are.
5. They don't need fancy or expensive; they just need your love and time.
6. Slow down and be present. Take time each day to release your to-do list.
7. You play, too. Rediscover your own "funtaneous" spirit. It's contagious.
8. Environment is the third parent. Make your home a peaceful haven.
9. Go outside. Nature is transformative.
10. Give children space and time to grow.

CHAPTER NINE

Love's Lasting Legacy

There are only two ways to live your life. One is as though nothing is a miracle.

The other is as if everything is.

—Albert Einstein

One night, after a dinner party she had planned with care, a Rocky Mountain mama started wondering if she had things backward.

"I would take time to prepare a wonderful meal, buy flowers, and light candles—for company," Lisa said.

Why didn't she put the same effort into family dinners? she wondered. There was no one she loved feeding more than her husband and children, so why was she relegating them to leftovers and pizza? Obviously she couldn't throw them a party every night, but maybe sometimes.

That's how the family dinner party was born. Now, anytime Lisa's husband or one of their children hits a milestone, the occasion is marked with a special meal and a little pomp and circumstance. Invitations are placed on everyone's pillow. Favorite foods and flowers fill the table. Party music sets the tone. Scattered candles create intimacy. Everything just feels special.

Family traditions and rituals create a sense of identity. Being part of something unique makes you feel the comfort of belonging. It's like being part of a school, team, or community. You know what you stand for, and you have pride in it.

We are the creators of our children's childhood. Make it personal with your own family rituals.

"A child with a strong sense of 'we' starts to develop a strong sense of 'I.'"

—Kim John Payne, *Simplicity Parenting*

Honoring routines creates the family "we" and gives children predictability. Knowing what to expect makes them feel secure. But in today's frenzied culture, unpredictability has become the norm. Payne writes about the importance of restoring a sense of routine and rhythm at home. Try to bookend your children's day with a soothing ritual. A regular rate and rhythm are the sounds of a healthy heartbeat. An irregular heartbeat throws your whole system off-kilter. Offer a regular rhythm in your home.

"I was always very conscious of the routines in my home. After a while, routine becomes ritual."

—Elizabeth, mother of three

And the ordinary becomes sacred.

If home is remembered as solid ground, people can reach further and withstand greater challenges. Family traditions lay down roots. The deeper the roots, the higher the tree can grow toward the light—and the more it can bend with life's storms without breaking.

MOMENTS MATTER

"Once a month, my family has a movie night. We all pile into my parents' bed with a giant bowl of popcorn and watch a movie. I can't even describe to you how much I look forward to it. We all do. I hope that I am never too old for movie night."

—Sixth-grade girl

Who would want to outgrow that? The family night she describes evokes warmth and coziness. That's what you're aiming for with family traditions—and parenting in general: closeness the whole family shares.

For centuries, that closeness came around the dinner table. But with today's schedules, family dinner gets squeezed out. Let's not let that happen. Family meals are important. Family time nourishes a child.

But it can be hard for that time to feel sacred when everyone is running in from different activities. One mom said hectic dinners with her boys felt like being descended upon by a hungry pack of wolves. T-shirts were used as napkins, fingers regularly replaced forks, and instead of having conversation, she was peppered with requests, spills, and interruptions.

So she reset the table culture. To gentle her sons, she would light a candle and have a moment of silence. Then everyone would go around the table and say one thing that they were grateful for. That simple change settled everyone down, turning her hungry pack of wolves back into little boys.

In homes with two working parents, family dinner may not always be feasible. But who said it has to be dinner? Several parents have turned to weekday breakfasts, and especially weekend brunches, as a realistic—and less rushed—family meal. So use creativity to make space for being a family and sharing food and stories.

You can also use meals to expose your children to different experiences. One mom wanted to share her desire to travel with her family, but she had no money to do so. Instead she brought the world to dinner:

"I invented international night. I wanted to share other cultures with my kids, other places that I dreamed of taking them. Four times a year we have international night. We pick a country, listen to its music, eat its foods, and pretend we are there." They all look forward to it and feel transported. What an adventure she gives her children without ever leaving her kitchen table.

Discovering more about each other can be its own adventure—if you ask the right kinds of questions.

"Family dinner was getting a little flat. We would ask our middle school kids good old parenting standbys like 'How was school?' and get monosyllabic grunts as answers. So I came up with Family Talking Teasers. Now we ask things like: 'If you were parent for a day, what rules would you

make?' Or 'If you could wake up in any country tomorrow, what would it be and why?' Or 'What's your idea of heaven on earth?' "

—Denver dad

Way to bring dinner back to life! Out went the grunts, in came lively, animated conversation. Sharing dreams with the people closest to you can bring you even closer.

Of course, after dinner comes bedtime. And bedtime rituals are the best.

Sam, a first grader, sleeps in the top bunk, above his brother. Every night, his dad calls from the bottom of the ladder, "Do you need covers up there?" Then he climbs up and splays himself over Sam, hugging him and asking if Sam likes his covers. "I feel so happy when he does that," Sam said.

Kids soak up intimacy.

"My dad crawls into bed with me and puts the covers over our heads and reads to me with his flashlight. That is how I know he loves me so much."

—Max, first grader

Rituals offer comfort even when parents can't be home to tuck you in.

"I'll never forget when my mom would go visit her parents in Florida, she would smack on her unforgettable red lipstick and kiss my sister's and my hand when we were asleep. We woke up with this big, fat kiss mark on our hands.

"Of course, this was in elementary school when it wasn't

lame to have a lipstick kiss from your mom. We quickly learned that if we were careful while washing our hands and taking showers, the lipstick stain would stay on for a few days. Every time we missed our mom, she was right there, and she always came home before it was entirely gone.

"It was just a little something, but it meant the world."

—Rachel, seventeen, Arizona

Leave an imprint on your children so they know they are loved. They will carry it with them always. On the other hand, if you don't engrave your love on their hearts, they will feel its absence.

I was struck in a family therapy session when a daughter cried to her mother that she never knew her mom really loved her. The mom was completely astonished and said that she had sacrificed so much for her daughter. But because her mother wasn't affectionate, and didn't say the words, the girl never felt how much she really was loved.

Give voice to your love. Demonstrate it with your actions.

"I know that my children will never doubt my unconditional love for them. But, more important, I want them to feel and see my love. And whether it is a reassuring smile, a listening ear, a really good hug or a kiss, I want them to know the joy I feel every time they come through the door."

—Richard, East Coast dad

Carol, a writer, made a "love box" for her six-year-old daughter. She painted Shari's name on it and decorated it with pictures of the things Shari loved. Any time Carol felt inspired, she would drop in a note telling her daughter how she felt. "I am so proud of the kind girl you are becoming." "I was so moved when you worried about the bird with the broken wing." "It's such a kick to be your mom."

Lucky Shari, to grow up with an emotional piggy bank filled with tangible reminders of her mother's love.

A Virginia dad made an annual tradition out of similar declarations to his daughter. On each of her birthdays, he would chronicle the depths of his love in a letter.

The first letter read: "Dear Andrea, I never knew what love was—until now."

By the time Andrea got married, her father had amassed twenty-eight years of love letters, and presented them to her in a book. Her wedding day letter read: "I am so thrilled that you found a husband who loves you so deeply. But I can assure you that he is not the first guy to fall in love with you. That was me, the very first time I held you in my arms."

I am not one to gamble, but I would bet that having a father who so freely expressed his love led the daughter to pick a husband who would cherish her as well. Putting pen to paper is a great way to reinforce your love.

"When my son was very little I started wrapping his birthday presents in homemade paper. I would write 'Paul, Happy Seventh Birthday' and describe the qualities he possessed: 'You are so kind/funny/sensitive.' I always felt really good about the paper. The toy or video game he would soon outgrow, but sharing my love was a tradition we both enjoyed, and it felt more lasting.

"When he got to high school, I wondered if he was getting too old for the 'I love you' wrapping paper, but since he never protested, I quietly continued. Years later I was helping pack Paul up for college. I reached up to grab a sweatshirt on the top shelf of his closet, and out fell all the years of homemade wrapping paper. I had no idea that he had saved it! I cried and he wrapped his giant, grown-up arms around me and hugged me tight."

—Midwestern mom

This mother took the time to craft words so meaningful, her son couldn't bear to crumple them up and throw them away. He held on to them—and her love—even as he went off to college. These are the best gifts to give your children.

And the gifts they give you? What you do with them can reveal your kids' importance in your life.

In her dining room, one imaginative mom has a large display case. Instead of spotlighting fancy china, Rashna chooses to showcase treasured children's drawings, paintings, and poems:

"I thought it would feel good to see their art and words every time I passed by the cabinet."

By putting the focus on her kids' creations instead of on expensive art objects, Rashna sent a powerful message to her children about what she values most.

Sally, a New Jersey grandmother, showed her family that she valued service and kindness above all. She told them she didn't want any more Christmas presents. Instead she asked her children and grandchildren each to perform a random act of kindness, take a picture of it, and write her a letter about it.

Those letters and pictures line her hallway, a daily reminder of the generosity of her children and her grandchildren. Now, that's a beautiful legacy.

OPEN UP TO OPTIMISM

As a psychiatrist, I often struggle to help my patients raise a low ceiling their parents installed. Each *you can't*, *you won't*, *you shouldn't* makes the roof and walls cave in, closing children off from possibility and dreams. Wouldn't you rather lift the ceiling so your children can see their unlimited potential? That doesn't mean propping your kids up with false praise. It means instilling a positive outlook, a belief that they can do—and weather—anything.

Jackie, mother of three, said, "I gave my kids the message: life is going to be hard. There will be storms, so wear your rain boots and take your umbrella or you will get soaked. Then, by all means, don't forget to wait for the rainbow."

You are the prism through which your children will see the world. If all you see are the storms and the gray, their views will be clouded by pessimism. But if you can teach them that sunshine is always on the horizon, then even in life's emotional storms, they'll know they can count on brighter days returning.

Years of research by Martin Seligman, the founder of positive psychology, shows that optimistic people understand that bad things are temporary and that setbacks are not personal failures. Seligman contends that optimism can be learned. So teach it to your children. Mindful language and your own positive attitude are great places to start.

"I would always focus on the positive," Jackie continued. "If my kids got eight spelling words right, I would focus on the eight gained, not the two missed. I taught them that their best was good enough. Mothers should never be the hammer drilling down the nail. We are the elevators."

Some parents believe criticism is motivating. And it can be. But fear-driven motivation teaches kids to beat themselves up emotionally, which is destructive. Offering encouragement instead teaches kids how to have compassion for, and confidence in, themselves.

I know; it's not as easy as it sounds—particularly when you didn't have an optimistic parent as a role model. One of my patients, Megan, had been breast-fed negativity by her mother, and worried that she would pass it down to her children.

"When I became a parent, I vowed never to be like my mom, but I often felt like I was in the movie *Freaky Friday*, like I had changed places with my mom, or at least I felt like I was channeling her."

Megan cringed when critical comments flew out of her mouth toward her children. Through therapy, she gradually learned to replace harsh words with more encouraging ones. "It was like teaching myself a new language. Often I would stumble trying to trade negative, judgmental phrases with more nurturing ones."

Your children need a loving parent most when they are berating themselves. Resist the temptation to pile on. Instead lighten the load. Try to translate your critical instincts into something more constructive. Consider these options:

DAUGHTER: I can't believe I missed those questions on my test!
CRITICAL MOM: You should have studied more.
SUPPORTIVE MOM: I know you worked hard.

DAUGHTER: I should have studied more instead of watching TV.
CRITICAL MOM: I told you so!
SUPPORTIVE MOM: What would you do differently next time?

The child who hears only "you should've" will feel defeated and helpless. But the child of the more encouraging mother will feel empowered to come up with her own solution: "I did need a break, but next time I'll make it shorter and just watch one show instead of two." Great idea and great mothering. Help children find a way out instead of digging the hole deeper.

Choose words and actions that let your children know you are their ally. Encouragement says: "I see you, I feel you, I understand you. I am on your side." And it lets children see mistakes as opportunities to learn instead of failures that drag them down.

The world looks different depending on the lens you are given.

Colleen and her best high school friend, Ashley, took two trips to the neighborhood art fair. In the morning they went with Colleen's mom.

"I remember having a ball. The food was great, the art was beautiful, and we had so much fun that we wanted to go back," Colleen said.

So Ashley's mom took them in the afternoon. And, for Colleen, the art fair took a 180-degree turn.

"I vividly remember her complaints: 'It's so hot and buggy today. The art is mediocre, the food overpriced.' I felt as if I were at a different fair. It did not resemble the one from the morning."

In that moment, Colleen was so grateful for her mother's brighter worldview. It made the fair, and life, look so much better. And it showed her that optimism, itself, is the real work of art.

"My mom lived by the famous words 'Life is a ticket to the greatest show on earth.' And, as a result, we did, too."

—Adam, entrepreneur and big dreamer

"My mom always told me that I could do anything, and oddly, I believed her."

—CEO of an investment company

As parents, we are the keepers of our children's dreams.

"I was raised to believe I could do anything I wanted and that wishes could come true. As a young child in Illinois, I used to have a recurring dream that I lived in Texas, where, at least in my dream, there were lots of apple trees with petunias planted around the base. I would tell anyone who would listen, 'That's what it looks like in Texas.' Rather than correcting or dismissing me, my grandpa planted a twig with petunias around the base in

my backyard for my fourth birthday. Scotch-taped to one wobbly branch was a giant red apple."

—Debby, Oklahoma mom and executive

"My parents always gave me the idea that even if I was struggling, hope was waiting just around the corner. I really wanted to start my own construction company. Rather than telling me it was impossible, they told me I was the perfect man for the job."

—Dad and builder

Tend to your child's dreams and watch them grow. That's what Brent Green's dad did. Mitchell Green was a lawyer and a judge, and Brent's brothers followed in his footsteps. But Brent loved plants. When he was young, and his mother went back to work, she left him in charge of watering the plants. Not only did he keep them alive, but he also cultivated them, eventually taking cuttings, planting gardens, transforming their yard—and discovering his passion.

When Brent was in high school, Mitchell sat him down to talk about what he wanted to do with his life. Brent replied automatically that he was going to follow the family path and become a lawyer.

"But, Brent, what about your love of plants?" Mitchell asked.

Brent said he could always garden on the weekend, as a hobby. His father didn't think that was good enough.

"Why relegate the thing that you love to the weekends? Why not be a landscape architect?"

Brent was confused. Law was a safe choice—the family choice—and gardening didn't feel like a secure future. He never knew his hobby could actually be a career.

But his dad knew what lit him up. He recognized and nurtured Brent's passion, and opened Brent's eyes to the notion that you can do what you love.

Brent's love of all things green turned him into a successful landscape architect, who beautifies not only his clients' properties, but also the world around him. Each year since his thirtieth birthday, Brent has planted his age in trees in his neighborhood, turning what he called an asphalt jungle into a lush, green community. To date he has planted over four hundred trees—and helped his neighbors replace bars on their windows with bushes outside them. His neighborhood has turned into a real community, and the crime rate is down by nearly 30 percent.

All this because Brent's dad saw his son for who he was. By teaching Brent to follow his heart, Mitchell opened up a career path that brought Brent great success and satisfaction—and helped an entire community bloom.

"Open your heart, fling your hopes high, set your dreams aloft. I am here to hold your hand."

—Maya Angelou

KALEIDOSCOPE

"Whoever has not a good father should procure one."

—Friedrich Nietzsche

If you've been well parented yourself, let's face it, your job is easier. You have a loving template to follow, and you can tweak it to make it even better.

But what if you did not have the best parenting mentors? I can't begin to tell you how many times in therapy I have felt patients' heartbreak about what they didn't get from their parents. They say, "My mom was not nurturing," or "My dad was really self-centered," or "My parents didn't see me." Without good role models at home, they wonder how they will ever be able to be good parents themselves. But they can!

"I had a really bad childhood. My parents made some awful mistakes. We did not feel happy or even safe in my house. But, God love them, I am sure they did not set out to hurt us. Their own stuff just got in the way. I did not want to carry that pain and anger with me for the rest of my life, so I forgave them, and I forgave myself. I sent some love to the little girl who had to put up with all of that—and then I made a decision to mother differently."

—Tales from the couch

This is what I absolutely love about being a therapist: seeing people evolve, change, and grow into the best versions of themselves. Although I intended to be a child psychiatrist, I switched to adult psychiatry when I realized that you cannot fully help children without helping their parents. So many grown-ups feel ill-equipped to be parents. Many patients tell me, "I had an emotionally unavailable mom; I have no idea how to be different for my child."

That's when you have to open your parenting lens wider.

Don't let your history become your children's destiny. Find your role models elsewhere. Borrow other people's lenses. Shift in a bit of color from one, a bit of light from another. . . . Stack them up like a kaleidoscope.

Maybe you had a teacher who took a special interest in you. Or an uncle who brought fun into your childhood. Or a friend's mother who made you feel safe and cared for. Maybe one of your friends' parenting is exemplary, and you can borrow from him or her. Or you were re-parented by a therapist who showed you a different way. All of these people can become part of your composite parent figure.

"When I was growing up, I would eat over at my best friend's house. Mrs. Gold would say to me the simplest things with such love in her eyes. Even if it were, 'Please pass the salt, darling,' I felt her absolute grace. We did not talk that way in my family, but I knew that, someday, I would talk to my kids like Mrs. Gold talked to me."

—Mom of two

We all need a few Mrs. Golds—and other fragments of wisdom and grace—in our parenting kaleidoscope. That is why I turned to so many parents, teachers, and therapists that I admired—to share their wisdom with you. May all of these wonderful people inspire your parenting. May your kaleidoscope be touched with color and light. May you embrace the gifts of so many great parents here, and offer them as a blessing to your child.

This is my hope. This was my intention in writing the book that you have just read. I honor the amazing journey that you are on. May parenting take you to the depths of your capacity to love. May that love for your children illuminate the path to your highest self, and as they grow, you grow.

Parenting is just that—a divine invitation to be your highest self. Accept it.

Your children and your children's children will thank you.

Shrink Notes

Love's Lasting Legacy

1. Family traditions and rituals create a sense of identity and belonging.
2. Routines in your home create predictability and safety for your child.
3. A child with a strong sense of *we* starts to develop a strong sense of *I*.
4. Create your own family traditions.
5. Give voice to your love, and demonstrate it with your actions.
6. Teach optimism; instill a positive outlook.
7. Focus on what is right, not on what is wrong.
8. Install a high ceiling; support your children's dreams.
9. The way you were parented doesn't have to be your children's destiny.
10. Build your own kaleidoscope. Bring the best parenting you've witnessed in your life into your own parenting.

CHAPTER TEN

Out of the Mouths of Babes

Ask the young. They know everything.

—Joseph Joubert, French moralist and essayist

"Parents crack me up. They say 'don't yell,' but they yell. They say 'have patience,' but they lose theirs. They say 'don't lie,' and they lie. Kids just copy their parents. It's not the kids who have to change, it's the parents. . . . Seems like Captain Obvious to me."

—High school student

"If I were in charge for the day, I would make a rule to eat candy and ice cream and play video games all day. I would turn my house into a candy jungle with gummy bear floors.

I might get a tummy ache. I guess that is why I'm not in charge."

—Kindergartener

"Parents should be in charge because they know more, because they learned more. Just look at the size of my dad—he looks like he should be in charge. He knows how to tie his shoes all by himself."

—Five-year-old

"I think that good moms don't let their kids do too much electronics. It can get boring to stare at a box and click the mouse. It is more fun to go outside and explore and maybe find a real mouse."

—Nick, seven

"My parents always went the extra mile for my birthday celebrations. One year they pitched two tents in our backyard. My friends and I played flashlight tag and made root beer floats. My dad told us ghost stories that were way more funny than scary. In the morning, they served us chocolate pancakes in our tents. I am thirty-two years old and it is still such a standout memory. I can feel myself smile every time I think about it."

—Midwestern dad

"My stepdad, Steve, came to me at a young age. I was about six years old, and he knew how desperately I wanted to be an actress. I remember he interviewed me about my 'new movie role' at Pizzeria Uno in downtown Chicago. I remember looking in his eyes and I loved him for loving me as he did. He had the sparkle that one sees with love. Every tiny-to-big hole that I had inside of me due to growing up without a dad, Steve filled. I am a whole woman because of him."

—Paris, twenty-seven

"I did not make it easy on my stepmom, Michelle. I was so devastated when she moved in with my dad. I did not hide my disappointment. I did everything to push her away and make her feel unwelcome. She met all of my rage and resistance with a calm grace. She always took the high road. When she should have been furious with me, she gave me empathy and care. Some twenty years later, I might go as far as to call Michelle my favorite person. I had never known unconditional love from a mother until she walked into my life."

—Grateful stepdaughter

"When I was a little girl my dad would wake me up every morning with a kiss and a question: 'What did you dream last night? How do I help you make that dream come true?'"

—Deborah, sixty

"My parents always make me look on the bright side. I would like to give that to my kids one day."

—Will, eleven

"I grew up in a rough area—every house in my neighborhood has bars on the windows. No grass, just lots of concrete. My parents would take me every weekend to a park with roses. My parents would make up stories about how my sister and I were rose princesses. I loved going there. It was my parents' way of giving us dreams, making sure we would not fall into a bad track. They kept us close. They both worked but managed to stay so active in our lives. I am the first in my family to graduate from high school and the first to be going to college. I thank my parents for staying so close and for showing me the park with the roses."

—Annette, eighteen

"I called my mom when medical school was really hard and told her that I was going to change directions and be a teacher. 'Great idea,' she replied, 'you would be a wonderful teacher!' Then the next day, realizing that I had passed my exams, I decided to stick it out in med school. I called my mom and told her the news, to which she replied, 'Great idea, you will make a wonderful doctor!' With my mom you could not lose. Life would turn out sunny either way."

—Lynn, twenty-eight

"I was cradled in love. So I learned to love deeply and effortlessly. It is that simple."

—Marcy, fifty

"One of the highlights of my childhood came during a long car ride with my dad. I was a senior in high school and my dad told me that he was here for me if I ever wanted to share anything with him; that he did not want to push me, but that he was always available to listen. It was in that moment that I decided to come out to my dad as gay. After an awkward silence, my dad told me that he was here for me and loved me. My dad asked if I wanted to tell my mom at all, and if I did, should he tell her or should I. We pulled up to my house and I told him to go ahead and tell Mom, and that I would wait in the driveway. Minutes later, when I entered my house, my mom hugged me and told me that she was happy for me and proud of me for having the courage to be myself. I felt so completely supported. All I felt was a greater closeness and that I have amazing parents. I feel very lucky."

—Robert, nineteen

"My dad leaves early for work, before I get up in the morning. Every morning when I wake up he sends me a text. 'Good morning, Alexa, I hope your day will be great. I love you so much, Dad.' I think great parents let their kids know how loved they are."

—Alexa, thirteen

"Great parents know that we are children. We don't know everything. We are not good at everything. I wish more parents knew this. If they did, then they would not yell so loud at my soccer games."

—Fourth grader

"Parents should stay calm even when they are mad. If they can't do it, how do they think we will be able to? Duhhh!"

—Fifth grader

"I don't think parents should yell. It is scary. Parents are supposed to take care of us, make us feel good. I get my feelings hurt. Yelling does not teach kids anything. Oh, yeah, it does. It teaches us something—to yell."

—Third grader

"My mom yells at us and hits us. At home I feel scared and always on edge. I live with her, I am there, but I am not really there. I have pulled away to hide inside myself. One day, if I am a mom, I will never yell at my child. Because yelling can destroy who a child is. If you don't feel safe with your mom, you feel unsupported in the world. My mom was yelled at by her mom, and now she yells at me. I will talk to my kids one day with love. If you talk to your kids with love, they will be successful in life. Even though I am only sixteen, I know this."

—Carly, high school sophomore

"I feel ashamed when my parents yell. Just tell me the same thing in a soft voice. Then I won't feel scared and ashamed."

—Savannah, fourth grade

"My father has been the person that I have always wanted to emulate. From his work ethic, parenting skills, spousal support, stamina, and goodwill, my father's actions have set the bar. I am honored to have called him my father, business partner, best man, and best friend throughout my life."

—Billy, forty-six

"The way my father treats my mother communicated to his daughter a woman's worth. Thanks, Dad!"

—Kathy, forty-two

"My dad knows that my favorite colors are purple and yellow and that I hate olives. He knows that I like gymnastics and he even watches it with me on TV. I feel loved that my dad knows me so much . . . even the part about the olives."

—Mattie, eight

"My mother loved me deeply and passionately. There was something fierce about her love. She expressed her

love often and without bounds—ardently, humorously, spontaneously, or sometimes very quietly and gently. And it was so genuine, it felt like bedrock I could always stand on. No matter what happened, somebody thought I was the most amazing thing on the planet! That's pretty powerful fuel."

—Joanie, forty-three

"I love just about everything about my parents. Kids soak up their parents like a sponge. My parents were kind and nice. That is what I soaked up."

—Emmitt, seventeen

"Each time I asked my parents if I could try something new, they would say 'of course' and tell me that they thought it was a great idea and that I'd be terrific at it . . . and then invariably when I would come to them six months or a year later and say that I no longer liked it and wanted to move on, NEVER ONCE did they give me a hard time. They would simply nod their heads and tell me no worries. I now think back to what an amazing thing that was. I see so many parents put so much pressure and guilt on their kids to be good at something and stick with it. For me, to this day, I love to try new things and I go into each with a sense of excitement and confidence. I totally attribute that to my parents."

—Ling, forty-four

"My parents knew that they could trust me. They always gave me respect and trust and so much love. Who would mess with that?"

—Manuel, eighteen

"My parents treated me with so much respect that I learned to treat myself that way."

—Brett, eighteen

"My dad would surprise me when I was in college. He would take a plane from New Orleans to Boston and then drive two hours to Northampton. He would knock on the door to my dorm room and I would flip. He stood there, looking very casual, and beamed in his southern drawl, 'Hi, sweetheart, I was in the neighborhood and thought that I would stop by.' He made the journey look effortless. That is how he loved me, effortlessly and with abandon."

—Ellen, fifty

"On birthdays at my house, everyone goes around the table and says what they love about that person. I love when they say it about me."

—First grader

"Parents should get to know their kids, stare into their eyeballs and look at them. Really good. In their eyeballs."

—Kindergartener

"When I was in fifth grade, I used foul language to fill out a Mad Lib. I was ten years old and trying to make a cute girl laugh. The teacher appeared out of nowhere. I was busted. My mother grounded me for Halloween, which, as a ten-year-old kid, was devastating. The next day, two teachers made jokes about it in front of the whole class. It made me feel ashamed. After I recounted what had happened, my mother went to school the next day and talked to the principal and my teachers. She went to bat for me and insisted that SHE was my mother and SHE would be the arbiter of my punishment. It was amazing to witness the love my mom had for me. She was disappointed that I had done something foolish, but she knew I wasn't a bad kid, and she was not going to let these teachers kick me while I was down."

—John, forty-four

"I am ninety-two years old and if I close my eyes, I still can see the way my mom looked at me with such love, such belief in me, like I was some delicious dessert. I have carried that feeling with me all of the days of my life."

—Betty Jo, ninety-two

"There was something about being a family of two in the world of larger families that made us go the extra mile to make things special. On Christmas morning we would relish a long, drawn-out gift-opening enterprise: light a fire, turn on the tree, brew tea, open the See's candy, put on wonderful music, and let the deliciousness begin! We loved to give each other coupons: 'One kitchen cleaning from your daughter.' 'One picnic in the park.' 'One midnight cow-tipping trip.' Creativity and generosity were the reoccurring ingredients."

—Olivia, forty-two

"In the chaos that was eight kids—plus assorted friends and neighbors—my mom was an oasis of calm. I love that, as I get older, my smile feels more and more like hers."

—Ella, forty-seven

"I would sit next to my dad on a winter day and he would let me put my feet under his sweater. We would sit side by side, just being together. I can feel the peace of it, even today, some fifty years later. I felt unconditionally loved."

—Jane, sixty

"My mom goes to work every day with a smile on her face. She cleans someone else's dishes, she takes out someone else's

garbage, and she cleans someone else's toilets. She does this for my dream of going to college. I can't think of anything more loving than that."

—Michael, eighteen

"My dad put a major deal on hold on Wall Street to come to my college lacrosse game. Children never forget that stuff. Look, I am forty-nine years old and I am still talking about it."

—Peter, forty-nine

"When I was in elementary school, my mom—a working woman among a group of mostly stay-at-home moms—always made the effort to attend whatever school events she could to support me. But, of course, she could not make it to every one. When I was older, my mom expressed to me that she always felt guilty for not being able to attend with the same frequency as my friends' moms. I responded that she had given me the greatest gift by being the perfect example of the modern woman I hope to be. Her dedication to me and my siblings was not lessened by the demands of being a judge, but rather, was made all the more cherished. My love and admiration for her is immeasurable."

—Nicola, twenty-one

"My mother showed me that it's never too late to learn and you're never too old to grow. She learned to say that she was sorry in her seventies, and now she is a pro."

—Stephanie, fifty

"My father's love provided us with a legacy of security. His love was not intrusive but always there. When I walked in a room, he would light up."

—Sara, fifty-two

"Great parents listen with love."

—Seventh grader

"When I hear parents saying, 'You are so bad, I am so mad, I am taking away your toys when we get home,' I think that the mom does not love her kid, because love does not talk like that."

—Nate, second grader

"My parents taught me to think for myself. I have my own set of beliefs and I tend to disagree with a lot of what they say. I don't disagree because I am trying to be rebellious. Rather, I just think differently, and they encourage that. I don't have to be like them to be loved. My parents and I have meaningful debates over current events. While I am a Libertarian, they are generally conservative, and

rather than trying to tell me otherwise, they encourage my different way of thinking. They are usually glad that I don't conform to whatever they say and like, like most kids do. And, besides an unusually low allowance, I'd say my parents have done a good job in raising me."

—Jack, fourteen

"My parents always trusted me to make good decisions. I often made horrible decisions, but they were all me and I learned a tremendous amount from them."

—Charlotte, thirty-five

"In graduate school I burned my leg and foot severely. I was careless in the kitchen and some parts of the burn were third-degree. My mother had to fly to Chicago, drive me to and from the doctor, and eventually fly me home. I needed almost constant attention. Throughout this whole episode, she was never once judgmental or accusatory. I cannot imagine how stressful it must have been, but she only met me with kindness, love, and concern. I was actually an adult who did something stupid. I try to remember this when my children do stupid things and I am about to yell."

—Rukshan, thirty-seven

"I can tell my parents anything. They are great listeners. They would always talk to me about drugs and gangs and tried to keep me on a straight path, as the streets outside

are crazy. I always felt that I could talk to them about anything, even if most other parents would freak out. They trusted me. It made me trust myself. Parents should never stop talking and listening to their kids."

—Lucas, seventeen

"Every year for Valentine's Day my dad buys me heart pajamas and then he makes me pancakes. I feel so warm inside my tummy even before the pancakes."

—Audrey, first grader

"No family is perfect, but I feel very at home in mine."

—Grace, fifteen

"My dad works very hard during the week. On the weekends he makes a point of spending time with me. We go for a burger and ice skating. I notice other parents want so much time for themselves, but my dad makes time to be with me. I am so lucky."

—Andrea, thirteen

"Love is that my parents are so nice to me, they talk sweet to me, they think about me, they take care of me."

—Becky, six

I Feel Safe and Loved . . .

"When I am near my mom."

—BROOK, FOUR

"At home with my parents."

—JAMAL, FIVE

"When my dad rubs my back."

—ALANA, SIX

"When my dad lets me put lipstick and jewelry on him. My dad must really love me to let me do that."

—HEIDI, FIVE

"Around my family. They make me feel good when they hug and kiss me. That's the funnest part."

—FIRST GRADER

"When I was two and a half, my mother died of cancer. My father cut back his work hours to spend as much time with me as possible. Despite the tragic loss, my dad always emphasized the importance of having fun. When I was eight and had friends over, Dad decided that we needed to have a massive water fight. Half of the neighborhood came out to join us. The typical summer day turned into a neighborhood-wide water war. Mixed among the seven-to-eleven-year-olds running around like madmen was my thirty-eight-year-old father. He has always gone out of his way to make the ordinary extraordinary, and his playful spirit triumphed over the tragedy that befell us when we were young. To this day, I claim that he has been the best role model I could ever ask for."

—Andrew, twenty-one

"My dad takes me fishing. He stands up in the boat and tries to tip it over. We fall in with our clothes on. It is so silly. I know he does that because he loves me."

—Gavin, seven

"My favorite dad memory is when we would sail in our small sailboat together. For both of us, I believe, it was a time of great freedom. I remember the feel of the wind and the sound of the waves slapping on the boat. We were often just quiet together. I think this is so important in raising kids, to have times when you are doing something together, and

you can just do that something together in a comfortable silence."

—Terri, forty-seven

"I like going with my mommy to Lake Shrine. It is so quiet there. It is easy to feel love when it is quiet."

—Nicky, six

"The guy I wanted to ask me to prom asked another girl. I was devastated. To make matters worse, my mom was out of town for work on prom night. To distract myself from my sadness, I went for a run. When I came back, I found my dad in the family room, sitting at a card table covered in candles and Chinese food boxes from my favorite takeout. He had chosen two movies for us to watch together. The guy I had a mad crush on who did not return my affection? Long forgotten. My dad's loving gesture? Unforgettable!"

—Diane, twenty-eight

*"I grew up in Guatemala. People would commonly come to the door peddling things. My mom would always buy them, not because we needed them, but because she knew that the people selling them needed the money. One time, on Mother's Day, a woman and her child just would not leave. They just stood there at our front door. '*Tienen hambre? *Are you hungry?' my mom asked. The woman cried. My*

mom invited both of them in, perfect strangers, to eat dinner with us. That was my mother."

—Sonia, forty-six

"Faith was an important part of my family growing up. We read from devotions every night. One winter Sunday after church, a homeless man asked my parents for money. My mother said she needed the driveway shoveled and gave him money to go to the hardware store to get a shovel. The man never came back. I was so upset that he had basically stolen from my parents, when they had been so kind. But Mom was unruffled. 'Honey, he must have really needed the money,' she told me. My parents really lived their Christian values."

—Shannon, thirty-eight

"My parents stepped in when a man was yelling at a taxi driver at the airport. That day, I realized that one of the most important things you can do as a parent is to show your kids to stand up for what they think is right. I believe that, for the most part, having moral, kind, and generous attributes will lead to a moral, kind, and generous kid."

—Hannah, fourteen

"My mom was the best listener. Nobody shared my joy more. She is still the first person I want to call with good news and she has been dead for ten years."

—Cindy, thirty-eight

"My mom drops me off at the camp bus every summer and she tries to pretend that she is really happy. She says things like, 'I know that you are going to have such a blast,' or 'Camp is so much fun.' She says these things while the tears roll down her face. As I find my seat on the bus, I always think about what a great mom I have. I look out the window and she waves to me with a huge fake smile on her face, as she wipes her tears and her runny nose. I know that she loves me enough to put aside her feelings for mine. That must be hard to do."

—Sarah, thirteen

"My father's humility runs so deep that not only does he never seek credit, he shrugs it off when people try to give it to him. He has such a strong sense of who he is that he doesn't need to advertise what he does."

—Howard, forty-seven

"When I was in high school, I went to a party where kids were drinking and doing drugs. My parents had always told me never to get in the car with someone drinking, no matter the hour. Still, I was nervous picking up the phone to call my dad at one thirty in the morning. He answered perfectly: 'I'll be right there. See if anyone else needs a ride.' Not only was he willing to get out of bed in the middle of the night to take care of me without complaint, but he was looking out for my friends, too."

—Anna, forty-one

"When I was in fifth grade, I was bullied for a short bit. My mom volunteered to serve lunches in the cafeteria. It was odd that my mom was there every day for that month, as she had a full-time job. She would flash me a huge smile as she scooped mashed potatoes and brown peas onto my plate. Years later I mentioned to my mom how coincidental it was that she served food around the same time that I was being bullied. She flashed me that same smile. It had never dawned on me that she intentionally stayed close to me when I was hurting."

—Natalie, thirty-three

"My mom knew my weaknesses but focused on my strengths. When I was anxious, she was calm; when I was sad, she was comforting; when I was happy, she rejoiced. By doing

this she offered me everything a parent can offer. And because of that, all of the grace that lives in her now lives in me."

—Tina, twenty-five

"My parents are great because they always do as they say. A great parent should try their best for you."

—Shay, eight

Acknowledgments

To say that this book was a team effort would be a massive understatement. This book stands on the shoulders of all the outstanding parents, teachers, coaches, doctors, therapists, and spiritual leaders whom I have interviewed (not to mention all the wonderful children). Thank you for your generosity with your time and for your wisdom. I owe each and every one of you a huge debt of gratitude.

I would like to thank my enthusiastic and powerhouse literary agent, Jan Miller. When Jan is your advocate, you know you are in the best hands. Thank you also to Nena Madonia at Dupree/Miller & Associates, who gracefully guided me through the publishing process while simultaneously making it enjoyable.

When I met Karen Rinaldi, my insightful editor at HarperCollins, I liked her immediately. I knew that she got it—and that she was the perfect person to champion the project. Karen's editing was spot-on, making the book crisper and more timeless. Karen seamlessly pulled together all of the elements that helped make this dream a reality, and I am forever grateful.

Thank you also to the entire staff at HarperCollins, with a special shout-out to Jake Zebede for his care, support, and professionalism. Thanks to Shelly Perron for her thorough copyediting.

I am so extraordinarily grateful to my talented freelance editor, Becca Rothschild. Becca worked tirelessly throughout the writing journey, and helped to keenly hone my concepts and ideas. Her eyes on, and heart in, this book have enriched it incalculably. My heartfelt thanks to Becca for her deeply meaningful contribution and devotion to this book!

Thank you to Pam Hait for her savvy professional eyes and valuable input on this project, and to the Kohn sisters, who really can't be beat.

My gratitude to Joanie Wread, whose profound wisdom as a writer and mother has touched this book. Joanie is an invaluable asset to any writing project.

I'd like to thank my colleagues at the Women's Life Center at UCLA and at Reflective Parenting for their support and encouragement. I'm deeply grateful for your friendship and the way you help me grow professionally.

Thank you, Elena, for your amazing attitude, huge heart, and enormous support.

Thanks to Kathy Oh for your hours of technical assistance.

My gratitude to Ron, whose enthusiastic guidance is greatly appreciated.

I am so blessed to have such amazing friends. You have been my greatest cheerleaders and encouraged me before I wrote a single word. The degree to which you have gone out of your way to introduce me to people who could help and to talk up this project has been extraordinary. Most of all, your belief in me has meant the world. I cherish and adore you. It is impossible to imagine my life without your friendship.

Thank you to my kind sister, whose spiritual journey has inspired my own.

Heartfelt gratitude to my brother, whose passionate support of this project meant so much to me. Thanks for making this book and my life funnier. And most of all, thanks for the magic.

My deep thanks to my parents, whose endless optimism, enthusiasm, and kindness have been the most precious of gifts. These gifts already have been passed down to your grandchildren and surely won't stop there. Thank you for the song in my heart.

My final thank you goes to my amazing husband, the keeper of my dreams, who could write his own book on what it is to be an incredible partner. Thank you for your meticulous attention to every aspect of this project and helping me navigate the business of writing a book. You championed this project as if it were your own. My deepest gratitude for who you are and for your magnificent mentorship of our children. As the proverb goes, when I count my blessings, I count you twice.

About the Author

Robin Berman, MD, is a psychiatrist and an associate professor at UCLA. She is a certified Reflective Parenting group leader and a Simplicity Parenting group leader. Dr. Berman is a founding board member of the UCLA Resnick Neuropsychiatric Hospital. She lives in Los Angeles with her husband and children.